# the healthy college cookbook

# THE healthy College cookbook

QUICK.

CHEAP.

EASY.

**Alexandra Nimetz, Jason Stanley, and Emeline Starr** ***with Rachel Holcomb***

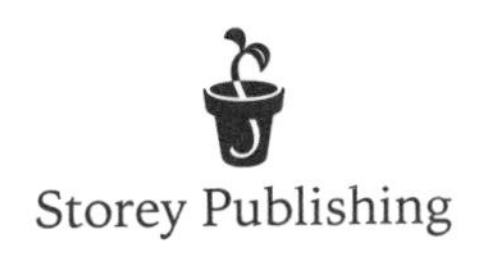

Storey Publishing

**DEDICATION** — To our families

*The mission of Storey Publishing is to serve our customers by publishing practical information that encourages personal independence in harmony with the environment.*

Edited by Margaret Sutherland and Nancy Ringer
Art direction and book design by Alethea Morrison
Text production by Erin Dawson

Illustrations by © Bo Lundberg [for Art Department]

Indexed by Nancy D. Wood



Printed in the United States by McNaughton & Gunn, Inc.
20 19 18 17 16 15 14 13 12 11 10

Library of Congress Cataloging-in-Publication Data
The healthy college cookbook / Alexandra Nimetz ... [et al.]. — 2nd ed.
p. cm.
Previous ed. entered under: Nimetz, Alexandra.
Includes index.
ISBN 978-1-60342-030-3 (paper : alk. paper)
1. Cookery, American. 2. Quick and easy cookery. I. Nimetz, Alexandra, 1977– II. Nimetz, Alexandra, 1977– Healthy college cookbook.
TX715.N683 2009
641.5'55—dc22

2008035261

## ACKNOWLEDGMENTS

While our names appear on the cover of this book as its authors, there are many more people who contributed behind the scenes to its ultimate publication. To those who contributed recipes, those who helped taste test our experiments, and those who offered support and help in other ways, we appreciate your helpfulness along the way. In particular, thank you to Amy Aloysi; Natalie Andre; Neal Appleman; Danielle Bahr; Allison Bergman; Meghan and Heather Brady; Alex Bresnan; Beth, Brendan, and Mary Buschman-Kelly, and Mary Kelly; Alison Cantatore; Tong Chen; Kip Darcy; Laura Davis; Maya Dehart; Rachel Dubin; Rachel Felsenthal; Katie Fogg; Mary Frekko; Lilly Gaul; Satie Gopaul; Lauren Greilsheimer; Anna Groskin; Peter Hardin; Matthew Karagus; Beth Lambert; Katherine Landry; Patti Lin; Tangee Mahdui; Sabina Menschel; Matthew, Gloria, Lloyd, and Meaux Nimetz; Dede, James, and John Orracca-Tetteh; Jon Putman; Sharon Rackow; Derek Sasaki-Scanlon; Emily Shanks; Frank, Paula, Bryce, Scott, Matthew, and Benjamin Stanley; Dan, Judy, Nick, and Dan Starr; Meg Turner; Kelly Virgulto; Victoria Wallace; Katie Wallach; George Warner; Christina Witter; Wells P. Wilson; those at Creative Gardening; and those whom we stopped along the road and in the supermarket to take our pictures.

Last, but certainly not least, thank you to Storey. Who would have thought that a brainstorming session in Pam's office during Winter Study '98 would have led to this? And thanks to Rachel Holcomb for collecting recipes from yet another generation of college students for the second edition.

# contents

# introduction

At the time of the writing of the first edition of this book, the three of us were all students at Williams College in Williamstown, Massachusetts, with no experience as professional cooks. Before beginning this project, we were like all of you: We often had no idea of what to prepare for dinner and really didn't have the time to whip up elaborate meals. This book was designed to answer your concerns and ours about how to eat healthfully on a tight budget, with a busy schedule, and with little cooking experience. We know that it's easy to settle for unhealthy food when you don't have the time to prepare something, but we hope that this book will provide you with alternatives to the evils of fast food. You can prepare many of these recipes in the same time that it takes to have a pizza delivered. We know, because we've tested every recipe.

For those of you who are especially health conscious, we used computer software to formulate a brief nutritional analysis of the calorie, fat, protein, fiber, and carbohydrate content of each recipe. There is also a section devoted to vegetarian and vegan recipes, but look through the whole book for the radish icon or the egg-and-null-sign icon. There are many options in several of the chapters.

The especially quick recipes — those that take ten minutes or less to prepare — are marked with a clock icon. If you live in a dorm room equipped with a microwave and a refrigerator, you will find many recipes that will work for you. They are marked with a graphic of bread and cheese.

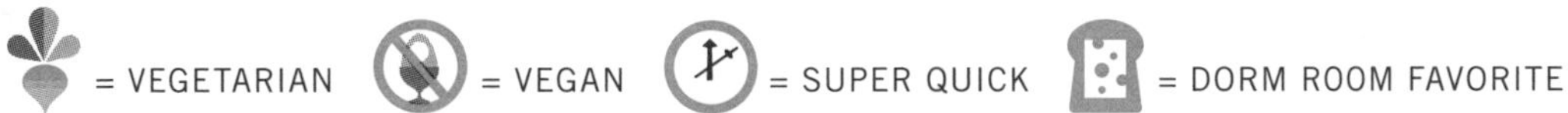

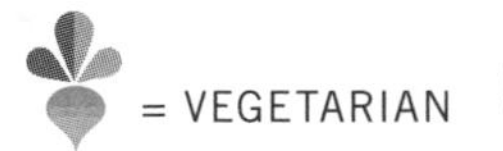
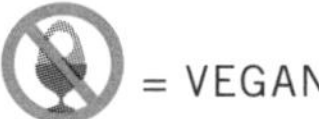

To all of our users: We hope that after using this book you will have a more solid understanding of cooking in general and will no longer consider it to be a tedious or unrewarding task. We have certainly enjoyed writing and testing.

*Good luck and enjoy.*

Alexandra Nimetz, Jason Stanley, Emmy Starr

Things have changed a bit on college campuses since the original publication ten years ago of *The Healthy College Cookbook*. There are more vegetarians and vegans, the George Foreman Grill is a big part of quick college cooking, and students eat more tofu and whole grains than in the past.

This revised edition includes 100 new recipes, submitted from college students all over the country. The original recipes are still mostly here (updated slightly in some cases), but they are complemented by recipes that reflect the tastes and ideas of college students now.

I hope you enjoy the new contributions, and I know you will find, as I did, that the old recipes are still quick and delicious too!

Rachel Holcomb

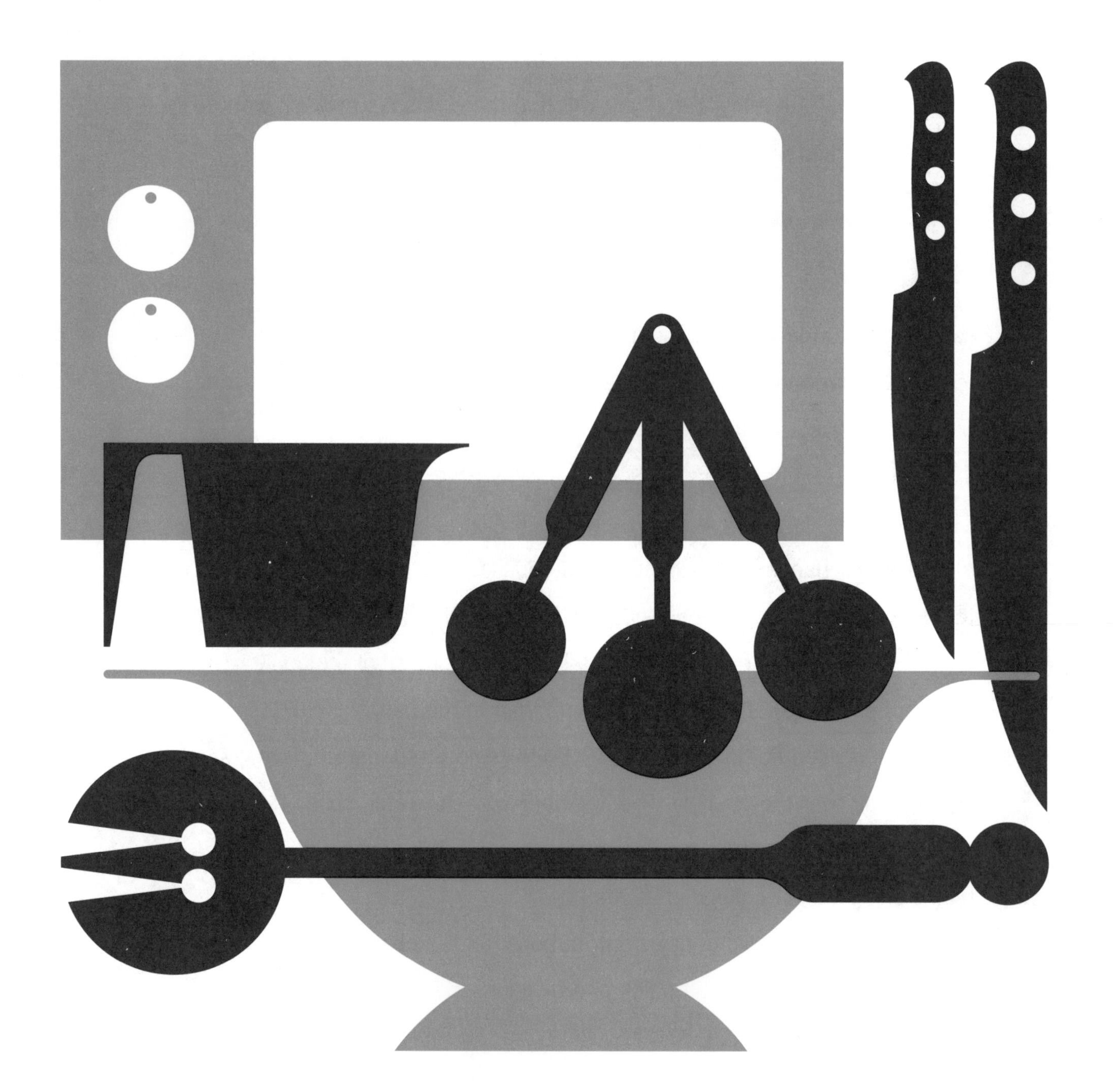

# chapter 1

## getting started in your first kitchen

Cooking is like any other activity: In order to be successful and have fun during the process, you need to have the right equipment. To that end, we've thought long and hard about the essentials for a novice cook's kitchen. The ideas and recommendations listed here will help you to develop a fully stocked and efficient kitchen — one that includes the basic cookware necessary for preparing our recipes. You'll also find suggestions for useful ingredients to keep on hand.

In the following pages, you'll find a glossary of fundamental cooking terms to read through for an understanding of the skills needed to navigate basic recipes. You will also find descriptions of common herbs and spices and some of their most frequent companions. In addition, we'll hand down to you tips that we've learned along the way, healthy substitutions for some not-so-healthy ingredients, and charts to help you to make measurement conversions.

We hope that you have fun with our book — we certainly did. Our most important piece of advice? Take your time, relax, and don't be afraid to get creative!

# setting up your kitchen

A bare kitchen can be intimidating for beginners, especially when it becomes obvious that you will have to equip your kitchen with some essentials. While it's not necessary to spend tons of money on top-of-the-line kitchenware, it is important to invest in the basics.

Shopping for your kitchen can be a tedious task, since it's not always exactly clear what it is that you need to buy. Sure, a pot, a skillet, and a mixing spoon may come speeding to mind, but what about a measuring cup or an oven mitt? To facilitate your shopping expedition, we have provided a list of items that we found, while making all of the recipes in this book, to be necessities for any kitchen. You may decide, based on your eating habits, that you don't need to invest in all of the items that we suggest. If so, this will not offend us in any way — each cook's kitchen is a bit different from any other's.

## COOKWARE

If you're lucky, you're moving into a furnished house with a fully equipped and stocked kitchen. For those of you who are not so lucky, the key to building a comfortable and functional kitchen is to give up dreams of endless stainless steel and Teflon-coated pots and pans. Instead, keep an eye out for the bargains. Buy cookware with multiple uses and organize your storage space (which, if your apartment is anything like the ones we've had, will be limited) so that the pots and pans you use most often are easy to grab.

In the interest of preserving your budget, keep in mind that you can usually pick up many of these items at yard sales or at a local secondhand store. This is especially true for the electrical equipment, such as microwaves, beaters, and blenders, which can be expensive in a department store but may cost next to nothing at a tag sale.

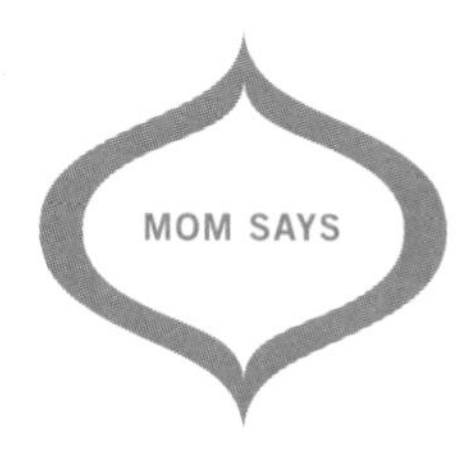


## hang your pots and pans

If you have a small kitchen, buy pots, pans, strainers, and spoons with loops or clasps for hanging. Install hooks (small nails will also do) in the kitchen walls and hang as much of your cookware as possible. It's an impressively efficient use of space that keeps the cookware easily accessible yet out of the way when not in use.

## cookware essentials

❍ **MIXING BOWLS**
You'll find that you need more than one, so buy at least one medium and one large bowl. You can use a cereal bowl if you need a small one.

❍ **SKILLET**
Look for a heavy, durable pan with a nonstick or stainless steel surface. You may want a couple of different sizes — we suggest a 7-inch and a 10-inch.

❍ **POTS**
Get one small or medium nonstick or stainless steel saucepan (in the 2- to 3-quart range) and a pot big enough for making large quantities of pasta or soups (in the 6-quart range).

❍ **CASSEROLE DISH**
Make sure that the dish is ceramic or ovenproof glass. We recommend having a usefully large one, such as 11 by 13 inches.

❍ **LOAF PAN**
We highly recommend having at least one loaf pan, as it is good for making not only breads but also smaller casseroles.

❍ **BAKING SHEET**
Buy baking sheets with 1-inch sides (sometimes called jelly roll pans). These pans are more versatile than true cookie sheets. If you're a cookie baker, you'll want at least two.

❍ **CUTTING BOARDS**
Buy two — one for cutting meat and one for everything else. Keep them scrupulously clean, as they can be carriers for food-borne bacteria.

❍ **DRY AND LIQUID MEASURING CUPS**
Buy a set of metal or plastic dry cups and a glass 2-cup liquid version.

❍ **MEASURING SPOONS**
Buy a full set and keep them separate from the rest of your silverware.

## cookware essentials, CONTINUED

- **GRATER OR MICROPLANE**
  Box graters are stronger than flat graters and less likely to collapse under pressure. Microplanes also grate hard cheese well and can be used to zest citrus fruits.

- **STRAINER**
  Strainers with "feet" that you can set in the sink are easy to use and clean.

- **SPATULA**
  Buy one with a sturdy head for flipping pancakes, removing cookies from baking sheets, and other such tasks.

- **CAN OPENER**
  You may starve if you don't have one of these.

- **WOODEN OR STAINLESS STEEL MIXING SPOONS**
  You'll need these for mixing and stirring. Wooden spoons won't scratch the surface of your nonstick pots and pans.

- **LARGE KNIFE**
  Buy a good, durable knife. Going cheap will cost you more in aggravation in the long run.

- **PARING KNIFE**
  A smaller knife is much easier to use for small jobs than the large knife.

- **OVEN MITTS**
  Buy two.

- **WHISK**
  A wire whisk is especially useful for making salad dressings

- **VEGETABLE PEELER**
  You'll be eating vegetables at some point if you think about your health, and this will come in handy.

- **DISH TOWELS**
  Buy at least three — one will always be dirty, one can be used to clean up as you cook, and the other should be left for drying dishes.

- **GARLIC PRESS**
  A good-quality press will give you fresh minced garlic when you want it, and you won't have smelly fingertips.

- **PLASTIC CONTAINERS**
  These will be useful for saving leftovers. You can wash and save the empty containers that held your cottage cheese, peanut butter, and other foods.

- **FLATWARE, CUPS, BOWLS, AND PLATES**
  You can usually pick these up cheaply at yard sales or your local secondhand store.

- **BLENDER**
  It's good for purées, pestos, and margaritas alike.

- **MICROWAVE**
  Although certainly not necessary, it does make the quick meal even quicker.

## STOCKING THE SHELVES

Now that you have equipped your kitchen, you'll want to stock up on some essential foods. As we've learned from experience, it's a common experience to begin preparing a dish only to realize ten minutes later, mid-recipe and mid-mess, that a necessary ingredient is nowhere to be found. We hope to help you to minimize the frustration and trauma that can result from these scenarios by providing a list of useful food items to keep in your kitchen.

We've presented this information in a checklist form to make it easy for you while you're shopping. While you may think that you'll remember everything that you need when at the supermarket, we guarantee that you won't. So don't hesitate to take this book with you. Just don't leave it in the cart!

### cupboard essentials

- ❍ RICE
- ❍ PASTA
- ❍ PASTA SAUCE
- ❍ CANNED DICED TOMATOES
- ❍ RED WINE AND BALSAMIC VINEGARS
- ❍ EXTRA-VIRGIN OLIVE OIL AND/OR CANOLA OIL
- ❍ COOKING SPRAY
- ❍ BOUILLON CUBES
- ❍ BREAD
- ❍ RAISINS
- ❍ CEREAL
- ❍ PEANUT BUTTER
- ❍ HONEY
- ❍ CANNED TUNA
- ❍ FLOUR
- ❍ SUGAR
- ❍ SALT AND PEPPER
- ❍ BAKING POWDER
- ❍ BAKING SODA
- ❍ VANILLA EXTRACT
- ❍ SOY SAUCE (LOW-SODIUM)
- ❍ ALUMINUM FOIL AND PLASTIC WRAP

### three easy odor beaters

1 Food storage containers made of plastic can absorb odors easily. To rid them of the smell, soak the containers in a solution of 1 tablespoon baking soda per cup of hot water.

2 To rid your microwave of bad odors, place a microwave-safe glass of water mixed with 2 tablespoons lemon juice inside and microwave on the high setting for 2 minutes.

3 To absorb odors in your refrigerator, keep an opened box of baking soda tucked away somewhere in it. But don't use the same box for cooking; those odors will be transferred to your food. Change the box about every three months. And don't just throw the old box away when the three months are up; to freshen a sink, pour the baking soda down the drain and follow with hot water.

## FILLING THE FRIDGE

The next space to fill is your refrigerator. Again, you will find that you probably want to start with some basics that are always useful to have on hand. Just remember, they have to be replaced more frequently than the canned goods in your cabinets.

### fridge essentials

- ❍ **BUTTER OR MARGARINE**
- ❍ **CHEESE**
- ❍ **MILK**
- ❍ **EGGS**
- ❍ **YOGURT**
- ❍ **JAM OR JELLY**
- ❍ **KETCHUP**
- ❍ **LOW-FAT MAYONNAISE**
- ❍ **MUSTARD**

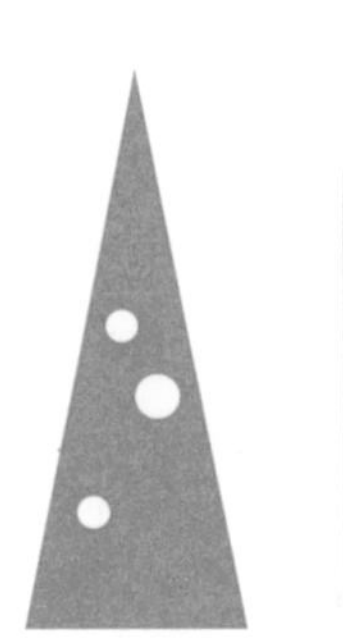

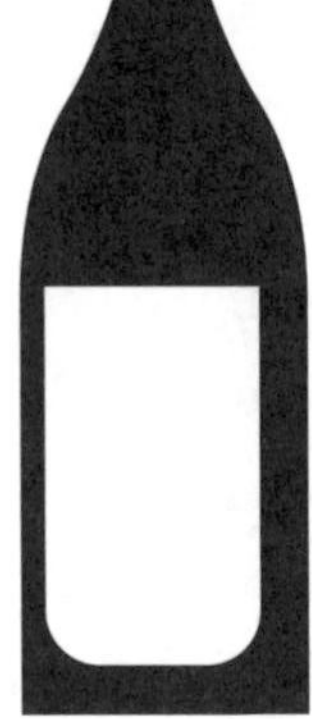

# understanding the language of cooking

Sometimes cooking terminology can be confusing. We have done our best throughout this book to keep terminology simple and to the point. Just in case, however, we've included a brief list of frequently used terms and their definitions so that there will be no misunderstandings. In addition to this basic vocabulary, we have included a few other commonly and not-so-commonly used terms that are useful for impressing friends and family.

## cooking terms

- **BAKE**
  To cook food in an oven with dry heat. Unless otherwise specified, always preheat your oven before putting your dish in to bake.

- **BARBECUE**
  Although barbecuing technically refers to cooking over a wood or charcoal grill, it has evolved to include just about anything — including roasting, broiling, or grilling — that involves barbecue sauce.

- **BASTE**
  The point of basting is to keep roasting foods, usually meat, moist by reapplying sauce, pan juices, wine, or whatever liquid you're using. You have all seen turkey basters, those giant eye droppers hidden somewhere in your parents' kitchen. They're used to suck up the liquid collecting in the bottom of the pan and dribble it back on top of the roast. Basting can also be accomplished by brushing or spooning the liquid onto the food.

- **BEAT**
  To rapidly mix ingredients. Should usually result in a smooth, lightened mixture.

- **BLANCH**
  The point of blanching is not to cook the food (usually a fruit or a vegetable) but rather to soften it, perhaps so that it may be peeled more easily or cooked very slightly. Submerge the fruit or vegetable in boiling water for a minute or two (the length of time depends on the food). It should soften and the skin will become easy to remove.

- **BLEND**
  To mix well.

**BOIL**

When you've heated a liquid to a boil, you'll see bubbles bursting up from the bottom of the pot. There are different degrees of boiling: a violent boil, a moderate (or rolling) boil, and a slow boil (simmer). Remember, a liquid is boiling only when bubbles are popping through the surface. It is not boiling when you see little bubbles resting on the bottom of the pot (although that means that you are close).

**BREAD**

As the name suggests, to cover with breading. Dip the food in raw egg or milk, roll it in breadcrumbs, place it in a dish, and bake. You can also bread with crushed cornflakes or potato chips, among other things.

**BROIL**

To cook under or over a direct, intense heat. Broiling browns the outside of the food and seals the juices in. You can broil under the broiler in your oven or on a grill. (Some ovens require that the door be kept ajar when broiling.)

**BURN**

If you are having success with this one, you probably should not be left alone in the kitchen.

**CHOP**

This dictionary definition, "to cut with an ax or sharp-edged tool; make chopping blows (at)," may not be the best suggestion for your purposes. The general idea is to cut into fairly small pieces. If you're going to be cooking the food that you're chopping, make sure that the pieces are all approximately the same size to ensure even cooking.

**CREAM**

To cream does not mean to add cream to a mixture but rather to fully soften an ingredient, such as butter, to make it creamy. When creaming, you will often have to blend in other ingredients, such as sugar, until the mixture is completely "creamed" or blended together.

**DICE**

To cut into very small cubes, usually about half an inch square.

**FRY**

Though fried food tastes great, frying is not usually considered the healthiest of cooking techniques. To fry food, break out the skillet and throw in some oil or butter. Heat the pan on the burner and then pop the food in. Be careful with hot oil; not only can it hurt if you're splattered (boiling oil will spit at you when foods, especially liquids, are added), but it is also a big fire starter if left unattended. See also *Sauté*.

**GRATE**

Technically speaking, to grate means to reduce to small particles — just think of grated Parmesan cheese. Using a grater will save you the trouble of painstakingly chopping and shredding foods into small pieces.

**GRATIN**

*Au gratin* is a French term meaning "browned topping." You can make anything *au gratin* by sprinkling some grated cheese, butter, and breadcrumbs over the top of the dish and then broiling it until golden. It looks good when finished and sounds fancy for dinner parties.

**MARINATE**

This takes a little while to do, but don't worry — you won't be doing much of the work; the marinade will be. Marinade is the liquid (usually flavored with various spices) that you soak a food in. The marinade will flavor the food while at the same time tenderizing it (if you're marinating meat). This will make cheaper, tougher meat taste much better.

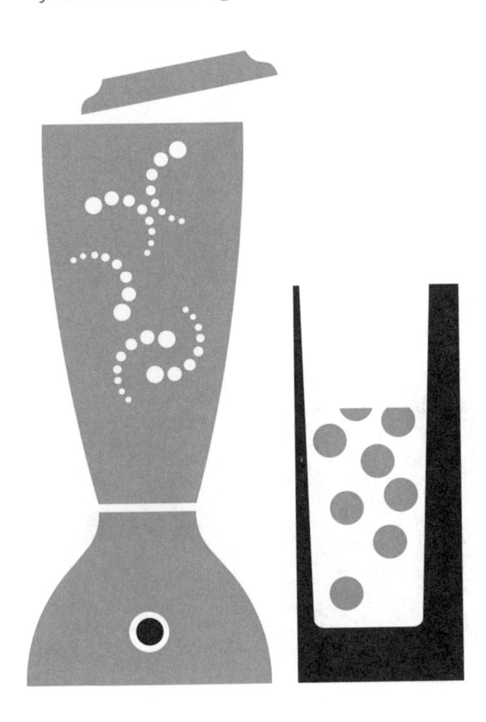

**MINCE**

To cut or chop into extremely ultra-small pieces.

**POACH**

To cook by simmering in a liquid that does not quite reach a boil.

**PREHEAT**

To set the oven or broiler to the desired temperature 10 to 15 minutes before use to allow time for it to reach the appropriate temperature prior to placing the food in to cook.

**PURÉE**

Remember baby food? Well, it's food that's puréed, so that it can be swallowed at that toothless age. Puréeing means putting something in a blender or food processor to make the food smooth and lump free. The blades turn and miraculously your solid food has a creamy consistency. You can also use an immersion blender, which is a blender on a stick that you can use to blend foods in a pot, rather than having to transfer them to a blender container.

❄ **RECONSTITUTE**
To rehydrate a dried food by adding liquid.

❄ **REDUCE**
Reducing serves to concentrate flavor while at the same time cutting down on the total amount of liquid. You reduce something by boiling it for a while uncovered. This causes some of the liquid to evaporate, leaving a substance with less volume but more taste.

❄ **SAUTÉ**
To cook food in a buttered or oiled pan. Sautéing is similar to frying, but it implies that you use less butter or oil and stir the dish constantly.

❄ **SHRED**
This slightly barbaric term refers to the act of tearing. You can use a knife or a grater to do it, and like in a paper shredder, the pieces should come out relatively thin and long.

❄ **SIMMER**
To simmer is to keep a liquid mixture at or just below the boiling point. You should hardly be able to notice any bubbles boiling up to the surface; the surface should just ripple a little.

❄ **SKIM**
To remove the top layer of something. For example, after refrigerating or freezing a meat broth, you'll notice a layer of hardened fat on the surface. Scoop it off and you've skimmed it. This is a good way to decrease the amount of fat in soups or gravies.

❄ **STIR-FRY**
To cook food quickly in a wok or skillet over high heat, stirring constantly.

❄ **TENDERIZE**
As you might guess, this term means "to make more tender." Some cooks like to gently pound some cuts of meat, thus tenderizing them before cooking or marinating them.

❄ **ZEST**
When you grate off the outer rind of a citrus fruit, you are zesting that fruit. You never want to include the bitter white pith when you are zesting fruit.

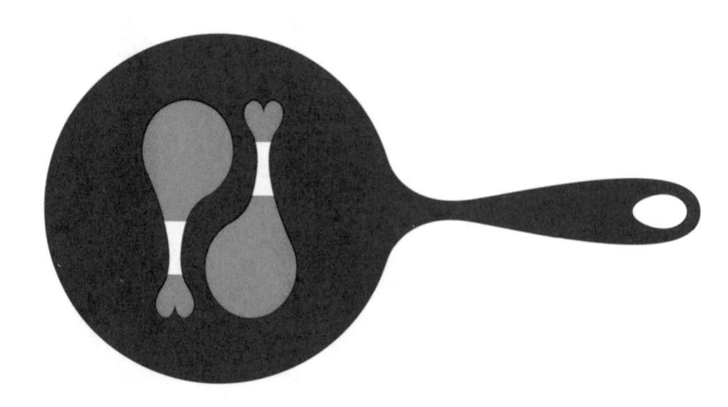

# herbs and spices

When we were first beginning to cook, our knowledge of using herbs and spices to boost flavor was pretty much limited to salt, pepper, garlic and onion powder, and cinnamon sugar. We figure that most of you are probably in a similar boat. Although we wouldn't think of going into great depth here — there are entire volumes devoted to the subject in every bookstore — we will provide an overview of the basics.

We are not recommending that you buy all of the herbs and spices mentioned in this section. That could be incredibly expensive. In order to preserve your budget but still have meals with seasoning pizzazz, we suggest that you invest in a select few herbs and spices. Our personal favorites are basil, cinnamon, garlic, ginger, oregano, and peppercorns. We've found that they are called for in a lot of recipes, and that with these six, you can find the right seasoning for just about any dish.

Dried herbs and spices come in small glass or plastic containers and can be found in your supermarket. Don't be afraid to buy generic-brand products. They usually cost considerably less and taste the same. If you have a natural foods store or cooperative in your area, you might find dried herbs in bulk bins or jars. You can buy very small quantities that will stay fresh until you can use them.

As for fresh herbs, there is no question that the real thing (as compared to the dried stuff) is far superior. However, when they're not in season, fresh herbs can be expensive or hard to find. So during the summer months, buy the more common herbs, such as thyme, basil, and cilantro, fresh from the produce aisle of the grocery store, but if prices go up when the cold season hits, stick to dried herbs. If you have a sunny windowsill and the inclination, you might even try growing your own herbs. Many grocery stores with potted-plant departments carry herbs.

Herbs can be fun to cook with when you gain the confidence to experiment with them. Start with a little salt and pepper here and there, and then try adding new spices. Pretty soon you'll be whipping up sauces and dishes that you never dreamed that you could create with your limited supplies. Just try to have fun with them, and you'll outgrow this beginner's overview before you know it.

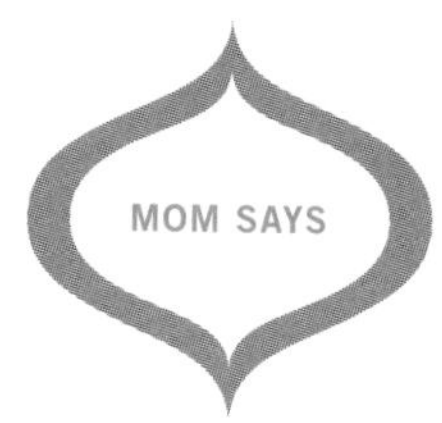


## dried versus fresh

In most cases, fresh and dried herbs are interchangeable. If a recipe calls for fresh and you want to use dried, use one-third as much as the recipe calls for. If a recipe calls for dried herbs and you want to use fresh, use three times as much as the recipe calls for.

## common herbs and spices

### BASIL

This herb is an essential for your kitchen and your life. If you have the patience for occasionally watering a plant and you enjoy the taste of fresh basil, invest in a basil plant; you can find them at farmers' markets, garden shops, and even grocery stores. You can usually buy bunches of fresh basil in your supermarket, somewhere among the vegetables. It is great in anything tomato-related, such as pasta sauces and tomato-mozzarella-basil sandwiches, and also in salads, pestos, and even eggs.

### BAY LEAF

If you've ever wondered why there was a big, crispy leaf in your bowl of soup, you are obviously not familiar with the bay leaf. It's commonly used to enhance the flavors of soups, stews, and chilis — dishes that require a long simmering time. It should be removed from the dish before serving.

### CAYENNE

For instant heat, throw just a pinch of cayenne in the mix. Also known as ground red pepper, it's great for spicing up chilis, burritos, stir-fries, chicken, and even guacamole. However, be careful when adding cayenne powder to dishes. Remember, you can always add more.

❊ **CHILI POWDER**

Chili powder is a mixture of ground dried chile peppers and other spices. The taste and strength of the powder depends on the brand that you use. Try sprinkling some in sauces, on tomato dishes, on meat, and, of course, in chilis.

❊ **CHIVES**

Chives belong to the onion family and, not surprisingly, have a taste somewhat similar to that of a young onion. Chives are often called for in recipes for soups, salads, and eggs. If you like cottage cheese, try cutting up some chives and mixing them in. It's delicious. Really.

❊ **CILANTRO**

Even if you don't know what cilantro is, we suspect that you've probably tasted it, perhaps in a favorite salsa. Fresh cilantro looks similar to parsley and is one of those herbs that people either love or hate. It has a strong taste that adds a fresh flavor to dips, soups, and, most commonly, salsa, including anything that salsa is used on, such as burritos or nachos. Use only fresh cilantro, never dried.

❊ **CINNAMON**

An extremely useful spice, cinnamon can be used in dessert dishes such as apple pie or in hot fruit drinks like mulled cider. Sprinkle some on buttered toast with a little sugar and you have a fast and delicious snack.

❊ **CRUSHED RED PEPPER FLAKES**

When you're looking for some extra heat for your food, add a pinch of crushed red pepper flakes. You have seen them in shakers at pizza places; they're great with any tomato-based food.

❊ **CURRY POWDER**

If you've ever had good Indian food, you'll appreciate curry powder. It is yellowish orange in color and, like chili powder, is a mixture of spices. Curry powder is good with rice, chicken, and vegetables.

❊ **DILL**

While the dill plant looks rather delicate, it has a strong taste that is excellent in salads of any kind, including green, cucumber, seafood, tuna, and potato salads. It is also delicious when used with carrots and fish (especially salmon).

❊ **GARLIC**

Garlic is great — in moderation, that is. Although it is typically associated with relentlessly horrible breath, it's wonderful for spicing up an endless variety of dishes and has quite a few health benefits to boot. If you don't like the smelly

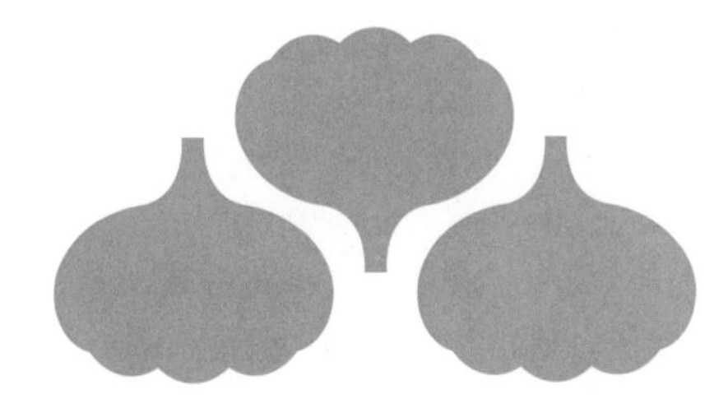

fingers that result from peeling and chopping the cloves, consider buying a garlic press, or buy prechopped garlic, which comes in a jar and can be purchased at any grocery store. Although garlic lovers and herb purists may wince at this suggestion, another alternative is garlic powder. It's cheap, requires no preparation, and doesn't smell.

❋ **GINGER**

As sushi lovers, some of us have a special fondness for this spice. Ginger is a root and can be bought fresh in the produce aisle of your grocery store. You can also buy ground dried ginger. We highly recommend that you buy one or the other, as ginger adds a terrific flavor to a wide variety of dishes. It makes a delicious addition to puréed vegetable soups and desserts or it can be mixed with some soy sauce as a marinade for meat, chicken, or salmon. If you buy fresh ginger, store it wrapped in a paper towel and sealed in a ziplock bag in your freezer; it will keep longer there, and when frozen it's easy to grate.

❋ **MINT**

Although typically associated with sweet dishes like fresh fruit salad, a few sprigs of fresh mint (or a few pinches of dried) are also delicious with peas and other vegetables. You can also use it in tomato sauces, especially those with meat, and it makes a wonderful hot or iced tea when steeped in water.

❋ **ONION**

The sharp and pungent nature of onion is mellowed when it is cooked. Onion powder is a quick and easy alternative, but as onions have a relatively long shelf life, we recommend stocking the real thing whenever possible and saving the powdered stuff for emergencies.

❋ **OREGANO**

Oregano is an essential ingredient of traditional Italian cooking. You can add it to just about any tomato-based dish and sprinkle it on most meats. It's pretty strong, so start with just a pinch and add more as needed.

❋ **PAPRIKA**

Paprika is a Hungarian spice that is made up of a variety of ground dried peppers. It is flavorful in hearty soups, sprinkled on top of meat or chicken, or mixed into spreads like hummus. As a bright red spice, it also serves to add great color to dishes — try sprinkling it on top of deviled eggs or tuna salad.

❋ **PARSLEY**

If any taste is "green," it's parsley. In restaurants, you'll see parsley as a common garnish for dinner plates. Use it chopped as a condiment for baked potatoes, and use sprigs tossed with salads or as a soup topping. Also important, parsley can help deodorize your hands and breath after cutting or eating garlic. Parsley is usually available fresh year-round — don't bother buying the dried stuff.

**ROSEMARY**

Rosemary has a very pleasant smell and is sometimes used in incense. It keeps very well as a dried herb and is particularly tasty with tomatoes, potatoes, chicken, and lamb. Try a stir-fry with tomatoes, chicken, a little white wine, and rosemary served over rice — it's simple and quick with a touch of elegance.

**SAGE**

If you can manage to use sage without getting Simon and Garfunkel tunes stuck in your head, you are doing better than we are. Dried sage is as good as the fresh plant and goes well with chicken, eggplant, and many soups and stews.

**THYME**

Like rosemary, thyme is exceptionally aromatic. Try it in stews or hearty soups, in vegetable mixes, and on meat or chicken. It's also pretty strong, so start with just a pinch and add more as necessary.

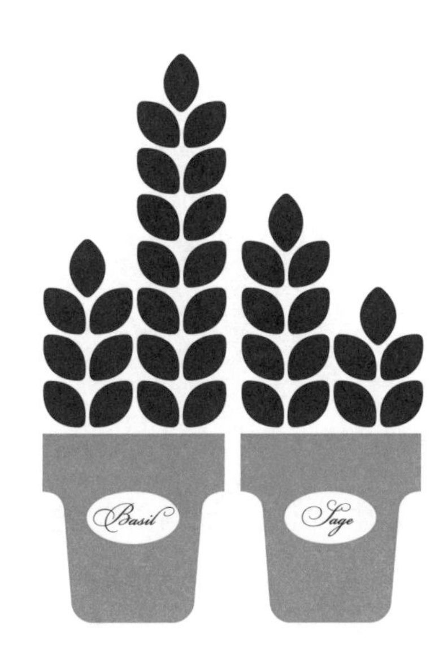

## authors' choice herbs and spices

These seven herbs and spices are essential for every spice cupboard.

- Basil
- Black pepper
- Cinnamon
- Garlic
- Ginger
- Oregano
- Sea salt

# complementary herbs and foods

The key to being creative in the kitchen is to teach yourself which herbs and spices create what flavors, and what they go well with. The following is a key to some of the most basic combinations. The mix-and-match ideas here will help you to develop quick meals.

## herbs for vegetables

| | |
|---|---|
| Asparagus | Lemon juice, dry mustard, or thyme |
| Broccoli | Lemon juice, dill, or garlic |
| Brussels sprouts | Lemon juice; white-wine vinegar with dry mustard and/or dill |
| Cabbage | Lemon juice; white-wine vinegar with dry mustard and/or oregano |
| Carrots | Honey, maple syrup, thyme, or dill |
| Cauliflower | Parsley and nutmeg; dill and tarragon |
| Corn | Garlic; onion and paprika |
| Eggplant | Thyme, garlic, or oregano |
| Green beans | Garlic, onion, or dill |
| Lima beans | Onions and sage; lemon juice and parsley |
| Mushrooms | Garlic, onion, or basil |
| Peas | Rosemary, thyme, or mint |
| Potatoes | Onion, garlic, and/or rosemary |
| Sweet potatoes | Nutmeg or cinnamon |
| Tomatoes | Basil and garlic; chives |
| Winter squash | Brown sugar, maple syrup, nutmeg, or ginger |

## herbs for meats

In addition to salt and pepper, try some of the following:

| | |
|---|---|
| Beef | Allspice, basil, cayenne, chili powder, cloves, garlic, onion, oregano, paprika, parsley, rosemary, or thyme |
| Eggs | Basil, chives, onion, tarragon, or thyme |
| Fish | Basil, chives, dill, parsley, rosemary, tarragon, or thyme |
| Lamb | Garlic, mint, onion, oregano, parsley, rosemary, sage, or thyme |
| Poultry | Basil, curry powder, garlic, rosemary, sage, or thyme |

# healthy substitutions

We suggest these substitutions, especially in baking, to make your treats just a little bit lighter. Remember to use them in moderation — replacing all of the oil and butter in a recipe with yogurt and applesauce will often leave you with a heavy brick. Use these substitutions wisely and you will find that you can't even tell the difference.

1 egg = 2 egg whites = ¼ cup egg substitute
1 unit butter or oil = 1 unit applesauce
1 unit butter or oil = 1 unit plain yogurt
1 unit mayonnaise = 1 unit plain yogurt
1 cup sour cream (in baking) = 1 cup milk + 1 tablespoon lemon juice (let stand 5 minutes)
1 ounce baking chocolate = 3 tablespoons unsweetened cocoa powder + 1 tablespoon oil
**And remember,**
1 slice chocolate cake = 27 minutes on the Stairmaster!

## helpful hints

After testing all of the recipes in the book, we have learned quite a few tips and tricks. To give you a jump-start, we've written up some of the tips that we have found most useful.

### SHOPPING

- Make a list of everything you need before leaving home. This is a good idea for a couple of reasons: First, you won't forget anything, and second, you'll be less likely to add unnecessary and costly items to your cart.
- Check expiration dates. This is especially important for dairy, meat, and seafood products.
- Stores usually place fresher foods behind or under older items. It's okay to rummage a bit — don't make too much of a mess, though.
- If you have a fish counter or a butcher in your supermarket, look at the specials there. Meat and fish ordered from the butcher or fishmonger are likely to be fresher and sometimes less expensive than prepackaged items.
- Try to avoid buying chicken or fish on Sundays. Some supermarkets don't receive shipments over the weekend, so you won't get the freshest product.
- Never buy dented or bulging cans. Dents increase the possibility of bacterial growth.
- When buying eggs, always open the carton and check to see that they aren't cracked. Aside from being a waste of money and a mess, raw eggs can carry bacteria that you don't want smeared over everything else that you've bought.

### COOKING

- We've all learned that the easiest way to make mistakes is by not reading the instructions carefully. This includes cooking. Before you begin, read the entire recipe.
- When using a microwave oven, make sure that all items put inside are microwave-safe. Never use aluminum foil or anything that has metal on it in the microwave.
- Don't use clear plastic containers to reheat anything tomato-based in the microwave — you'll end up with all of your containers stained red. In fact, some health practitioners argue that, when microwaved, soft plastic containers leak toxic substances into the food they contain, so you may want to consider using just regular (but microwave-safe) plates and bowls in the microwave.

- Make sure that there are no paper, plastic, or other flammable items near the stove.
- When cooking on the stovetop, never leave the handles of pots or pans turned outward. Turning the handles to the side eliminates the chance that you or hungry, impatient friends walking past the stove will accidentally knock them off.
- Always remember to stir, especially when reheating. If you don't, things that have settled to the bottom of the pot will burn.
- Always check twice to make sure that the oven and stove are off — you don't want to burn the place down.

## FREEZING

- Label items before freezing them. We guarantee that no matter how in touch you think you are with the contents of your freezer, at some point everything will begin to look the same.
- When preparing dishes for freezing, think ahead and wrap up portions in the quantities you will want to thaw. For example, in order to save yourself the time and trouble of defrosting a whole block of ground beef, mold the beef into single-serving patties before freezing. This way you can defrost only what you need.
- Make sure that items placed in the freezer are wrapped well. Bags or containers need to be airtight to prevent freezer burn.
- Prep all items exactly as you want them before freezing. For example, before freezing chicken, remove the fatty parts. You'll save yourself time later.

## DEFROSTING

- Use a microwave for defrosting. It's simple and efficient. Make sure you remove any aluminum foil or plastic wrap first.
- Do not defrost any dish that, when fresh, needs to be refrigerated (such as dishes containing fish, poultry, or meat) by leaving it out at room temperature — keep it in the refrigerator. The outer parts, which defrost much more quickly than the inner parts, can easily go bad if left out.
- Plan ahead. If you're going to have to defrost something for dinner, take it out of the freezer the night or morning before and put it into the refrigerator. It will be defrosted, or at least mostly defrosted, by the time you want to cook it.
- Keep items that are defrosting on a plate. As they defrost, frozen foods leak a lot of water, which can make quite a mess if you don't prepare for it.
- Use cuts of fish, poultry, or meat within 24 hours of defrosting them. Never refreeze these items.

## REHEATING

- Using a microwave is probably the simplest way to reheat food. Remember to stir occasionally, since a microwave won't heat the food uniformly. If your microwave does not rotate the food while heating, be sure to do so yourself.
- When reheating on a stovetop, use a low flame or low heat to maintain consistency and prevent burning. Stir frequently.

## HANDLING MEATS

- Always rinse raw poultry with cold water before using it.
- Try to minimize the amount of contact raw meat (including fish and poultry) has with anything in the kitchen, including countertops, cutting boards, knives, and plates. Wash those items thoroughly with hot water and soap before using them again.
- When cooking chicken or pork, you must make sure that it is completely done. This means no pink inside. When in doubt, cook longer.
- If you've bought a package of meat but you don't need all of it for your recipe, it's a good idea to cook it all anyway. You can always use the cooked meat in the next dish you prepare. If you don't cook it, freeze the remainder. It can spoil quickly if left in an open package in the refrigerator.

## CLEANING UP

- Don't let dishes pile up. The longer you let them go, the harder it will be to get them done.
- Clean up as you go. While your dish is simmering, it doesn't require much of your attention. Use this opportunity to get a jump on the cleaning. Put spices back on the shelf. Wash the silverware, bowls, and pots that you've used. Even though you may get them messy again, wipe down the counters — it's easier and more pleasant to cook in a clean kitchen. In addition to saving you time in the long run, you'll find it easier to be motivated and do the less pleasant chores before you get full and slide into a food coma.
- If you have to clean an especially hard-to-scrub pan, first fill it with hot water and dishwashing soap and let it soak for a few hours.
- When cleaning dishes, use hot water. It helps to break down the oils.
- Always clean counters and stovetops after cooking. It's a two-minute task that makes the kitchen look a million times cleaner and will make cooking the next time a much more appealing job.

# helpful conversions

We have listed ingredients for our recipes in standard measurements, but we have found it convenient to have a metric index that you can call on when cooking. In addition, the conversions listed here are also a breakdown of the units in the standard system.

## weight

1 ounce........................28.5 grams
¼ pound ........................ 113 grams
½ pound ........................225 grams
1 pound (16 ounces) .....450 grams

## volume

1 teaspoon ..............................5 ml
1 tablespoon (3 teaspoons)....15 ml
¼ cup (4 tablespoons) ...........60 ml
⅓ cup ...................................80 ml
½ cup (8 tablespoons)..........125 ml
1 cup (8 fluid ounces)..........250 ml
2 cups (16 fluid ounces) ..... 500 ml
4 cups (1 quart)................1,000 ml

## temperature

To quickly convert centigrade into Fahrenheit, multiply by 9, divide by 5, and add 32. To convert Fahrenheit into centigrade, subtract 32, multiply by 5, and divide by 9.

32°F ..................0°C (freezing point of water)
100°F ................38°C
212°F .............. 100°C (boiling point of water)
325°F .............. 163°C
350°F .............. 177°C
375°F ...............191°C
400°F ..............204°C
425°F .............. 218°C
450°F ..............232°C

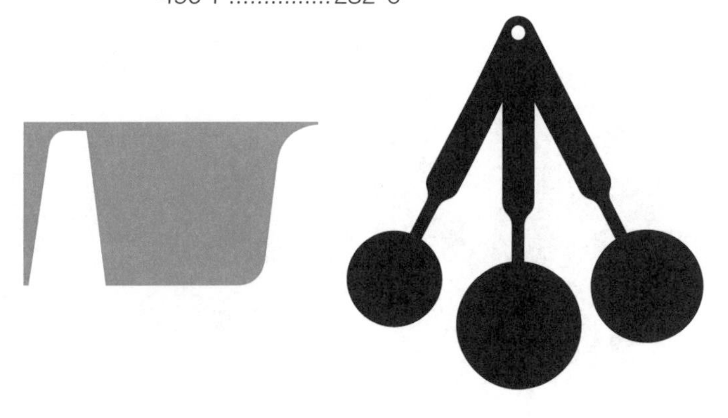

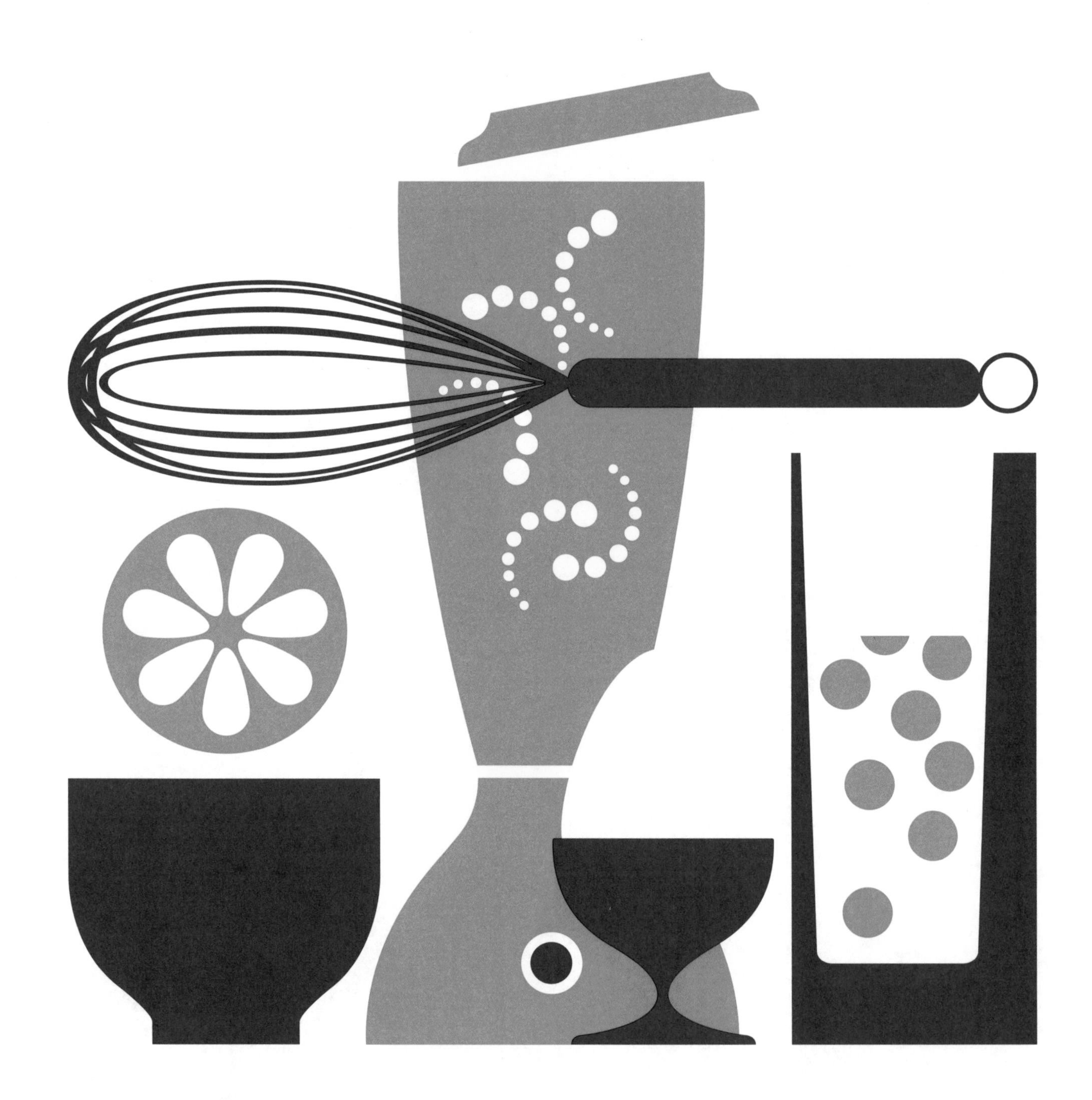

# chapter 2

## champion breakfasts

Everyone has heard that breakfast is the most important meal of the day. Breakfast kick-starts your metabolism, feeds your brain, and prepares you for what lies ahead. Among college students, however, skipping breakfast still seems to be a contagious disease. If you find yourself all too often running out the door with a rumbling stomach, we suggest that you take a look at the following pages. Some of the recipes can even be prepared the night before for those days when you know you won't have much time.

You'll notice that we've included quite a few egg recipes here. Egg whites are full of protein and have no cholesterol or fat. There are also plenty of high-quality, no-cholesterol egg substitutes that work just as well as the real thing in many recipes. With eggs, you can make all sorts of elegant dishes, such as omelets, quiches, and frittatas, quickly and cheaply. Avoid eating raw eggs — or taste-testing recipes that have raw eggs in them before they are cooked — as they can contain salmonella.

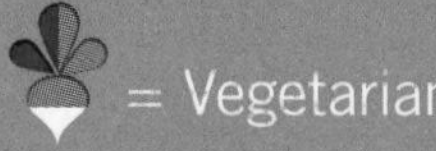


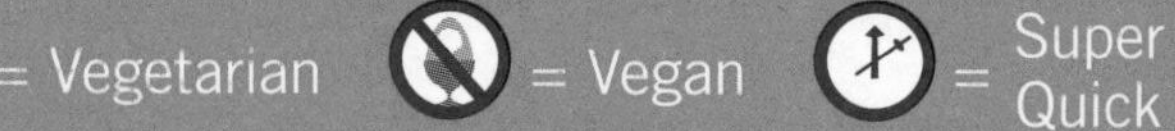


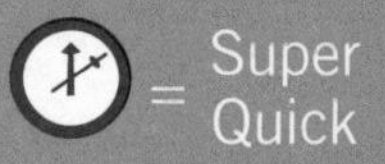


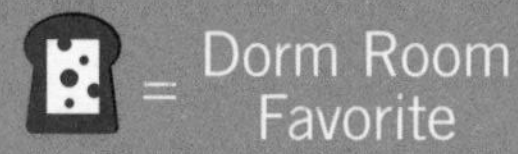

# cold fruit cereal

 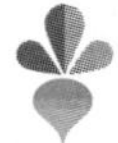 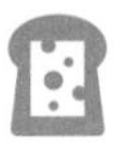

MAKES 2 SERVINGS

**¼ cup quick-cooking oats**
**½ cup skim milk**
**¼ cup nonfat plain yogurt**
**½ cup orange juice**
**1½ tablespoons honey**
**1 apple, peeled, cored, and chopped**
**¼ cup mixed fruit, chopped (optional)**

1. Combine the oats, milk, and yogurt in a medium bowl. Let stand for 5 minutes to allow the oats to soften.
2. Stir in the orange juice, honey, apple, and mixed fruit, if using. Mix well. Serve cold.

NUTRITION PER SERVING
Calories 200 • Fat 1 g • Fiber 3 g • Protein 6 g • Carbohydrates 44 g

# apple oatmeal

MAKES 2 SERVINGS

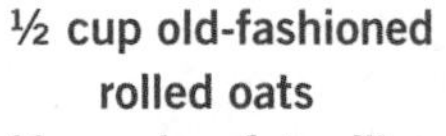

**½ cup old-fashioned rolled oats**
**½ cup low-fat milk**
**½ cup water**
**2 tablespoons raisins**
**½ tablespoon packed brown sugar**
**½ apple, peeled, cored, and chopped**
**Pinch of salt**
**Cinnamon for sprinkling**

1. Mix together the oats, milk, water, raisins, sugar, apple, and salt in a saucepan. Bring to a boil, then cover, reduce heat, and simmer for 10 minutes, stirring frequently.
2. When the mixture is thick and mushy, remove from heat. Sprinkle with cinnamon and serve.

NUTRITION PER SERVING
Calories 180 • Fat 2 g • Fiber 4 g • Protein 6 g • Carbohydrates 37 g

# granola

MAKES 20 SERVINGS

This recipe makes quite a bit of granola, which will keep for about a month when stored in an airtight container. Try it sprinked over yogurt and fruit.

**3 cups old-fashioned rolled oats**
**½ cup sunflower seeds, shelled**
**½ cup pumpkin seeds**
**½ cup chopped walnuts**
**½ cup chopped almonds**
**3 tablespoons butter, melted**
**2 tablespoons vegetable oil**
**2 tablespoons molasses**
**¼ cup dark corn syrup**

1. Preheat the oven to 400°F.
2. Combine the oats, seeds, and nuts in a large bowl.
3. Combine the butter, oil, molasses, and corn syrup in a separate bowl, stirring until well blended. Pour onto the oat mixture and mix well.
4. Spread the mixture in a shallow baking pan. Bake for about 15 minutes, stirring occasionally, until the mixture is dry and crunchy.

NUTRITION PER SERVING

Calories 150 • Fat 9 g • Fiber 2 g • Protein 4 g • Carbohydrates 15 g

## in the long run

This recipe may seem expensive when you go to buy the ingredients, but remember that it will keep for a long time in a sealed plastic container. Also keep in mind how expensive cereal is — in comparison, this recipe is a good deal *and* you're not eating all of those artificial preservatives and sweeteners.

## peanut butter oatmeal

  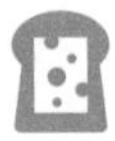

MAKES 1 SERVING

This is a filling comfort food after a long day of studying.

**½ cup water**
**¼ cup quick-cooking oats**
**1 teaspoon packed brown sugar**
**¼ cup peanut butter**

1 Stir the water and oats together in a microwave-safe container.

2 Heat the cereal in the microwave for 1 to 2 minutes, until the oats are soft. Stir in the sugar and peanut butter.

NUTRITION PER SERVING
Calories 290 • Fat 18 g • Fiber 4 g • Protein 11 g • Carbohydrates 15 g

## crunchy oatmeal

  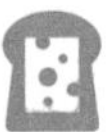

MAKES 2 SERVINGS

This is a delicious, warming breakfast — a great way to start the day!

**1 cup old-fashioned rolled oats**
**2 cups water**
**2 teaspoons cinnamon**
**Sweetener of choice (optional)**
**1 plain granola bar, crushed**

1 Combine the oats, water, and cinnamon in a microwave-safe bowl. Microwave on high for about 2 minutes, or until the oats are tender.

2 Divide the oatmeal into 2 bowls. Add sweetener to taste, if desired. Top each bowl with half of the crumbs from the crushed granola bar. Serve immediately.

NUTRITION PER SERVING
Calories 220 • Fat 5 g • Fiber 6 g • Protein 8 g • Carbohydrates 37 g

## traditional pancakes

MAKES 3 SERVINGS, OR ABOUT 9 PANCAKES

This recipe works for all kinds of pancakes. Try mixing in blueberries, apples, peaches, or even chocolate chips. Save any leftovers, wrapped in plastic wrap, for a late-night snack or tomorrow's breakfast. One word of advice: When it comes to maple syrup, it's worthwhile to splurge. There's no substitute for the real thing.

**1 cup all-purpose flour**
**½ teaspoon baking powder**
**2 tablespoons sugar**
**Pinch of salt**
**1 egg**
**1 cup skim milk**
**1 tablespoon vegetable oil**
**1 teaspoon vanilla extract**
**Cooking spray**

1. Combine the flour, baking powder, sugar, and salt in a medium bowl.
2. In a large bowl, whisk together the egg, milk, oil, and vanilla. Add the dry ingredients and stir until the mixture is smooth.
3. Heat a nonstick skillet over medium heat until a drop of water dances on the surface. Coat the skillet lightly with cooking spray. Pour small puddles of batter, one for each pancake, into the skillet. Do not crowd the pancakes. (If you don't have a nonstick skillet, you'll need to melt a little butter in the pan first to keep the pancakes from sticking.) Cook until bubbles begin to appear and pop on the uncooked side. Flip and cook the other side. When both sides are golden brown, remove the pancakes from the pan and keep warm while you cook the rest of the batter.

NUTRITION PER SERVING
Calories 280 • Fat 7 g • Fiber 1 g • Protein 9 g • Carbohydrates 45 g

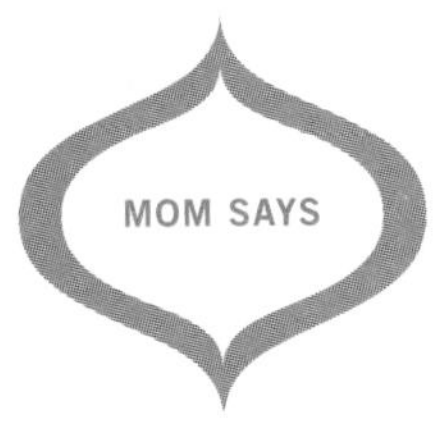


### while you're waiting

To keep pancakes warm while you finish preparing the remainder of the meal, stack them on a plate or baking dish in a 200°F oven. Place a paper towel between each pancake to keep them from getting soggy.

# orange cinnamon tofu toast

MAKES 2 SERVINGS

Tofu can be delicious for breakfast too. In this recipe tofu takes on the familiar morning flavors of orange juice and cinnamon sugar.

**½ cup orange juice**
**1 teaspoon cinnamon**
**1 teaspoon sugar**
**¼ (1-pound) package firm tofu, sliced into 4 thin strips**
**4 slices whole-wheat bread**

1. Combine the orange juice, cinnamon, and sugar in a medium saucepan over medium heat.
2. When the mixture begins to bubble, add the strips of tofu. Cook for 3 minutes.
3. While the tofu is heating, toast the bread.
4. Remove the tofu from the saucepan and lay a few strips on each slice of toast. Drizzle with juice from the pan.

NUTRITION PER SERVING

Calories 190 • Fat 5 g • Fiber 5 g • Protein 14 g • Carbohydrates 31 g

# orange french toast

MAKES 4 SERVINGS

Serve each person two slices of French toast with orange-strawberry syrup poured over the top. If it's just you at the table, halve the recipe or save the leftovers for later.

**1½ cups orange juice**
**2 eggs**
**¼ cup skim milk**
**¼ teaspoon cinnamon**
**½ teaspoon sugar**
**¼ cup strawberry jam**
**2 teaspoons butter or margarine**
**8 slices whole-wheat bread**

1. Combine ½ cup of the orange juice and the eggs, milk, cinnamon, and sugar in a bowl. Set aside.
2. In a small saucepan, combine the remaining 1 cup of orange juice and the strawberry jam. Heat to a simmer, stirring constantly, until most of the jam is liquefied. Continue to simmer over low heat until the mixture reaches a thick, syrupy consistency.
3. Melt ½ teaspoon of the butter in a large nonstick skillet over medium heat. Dip the bread (1 piece at a time) in the egg mixture, turning to coat both sides.
4. Cook each piece of bread in the skillet until both sides are golden brown. For each piece of bread, add more butter to the pan as necessary.

NUTRITION PER SERVING

Calories 260 • Fat 8 g • Fiber 5 g • Protein 12 g • Carbohydrates 63 g

# english muffin sundaes

MAKES 2 SERVINGS

As sweet and tasty as dessert but so healthy you can eat it for breakfast!

- **1 egg**
- **¼ cup skim milk**
- **1 teaspoon vanilla**
- **2 whole-wheat English muffins**
- **1 banana, sliced**
- **4 strawberries, sliced**
- **8 ounces nonfat strawberry yogurt**

1. Preheat a nonstick skillet over medium heat. Whisk together the egg, milk, and vanilla in a shallow dish.
2. Slice the English muffins in half. Dip each muffin half in the egg mixture, turning to coat both sides, and set the muffins in the skillet. Cook for 2 minutes per side until golden.
3. Remove the muffins from the skillet and set them on plates. Top them with fruit and yogurt. Enjoy!

**NUTRITION PER SERVING**

Calories 310 • Fat 4 g • Fiber 7 g • Protein 14 g • Carbohydrates 1 g

# hard-boiled egg

MAKES 1 SERVING

Many people have asked, "Just how healthy is an egg?" Eaten occasionally, eggs are a good source of low-calorie protein, and a hard-boiled egg is one of the quickest breakfasts or snacks that you'll find.

**1 egg**

1. Place the egg in a saucepan and cover with cold water. Bring the water to a boil. As soon as the water boils, remove the pan from the heat, cover, and let stand for 12 minutes.
2. Using tongs, remove the egg from the water and rinse it under cold water until it is cool enough to peel.

NUTRITION PER SERVING

Calories 80 • Fat 5 g • Fiber 0 g • Protein 6 g • Carbohydrates 1 g

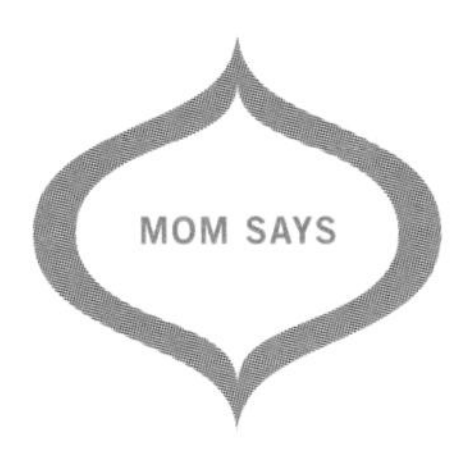


## buying eggs

- The natural shell color of eggs does not affect their nutritive value, flavor, or cooking performance. The color is determined simply by the breed of hen laying the egg.
- Remember to check your eggs before leaving the supermarket; don't buy eggs that are cracked or broken. If you crack an egg on the way home, use it within a day — no longer — in a dish that will be well cooked.

# scrambled eggs

MAKES 2 SERVINGS

Perk up your scrambled eggs with diced onions, peppers, or tomatoes. Sautéed, sliced mushrooms are also delicious with eggs. Or fold the eggs into tortillas with a spoonful of salsa and a slice or two of avocado for a portable breakfast wrap.

**3 eggs**
**1 tablespoon skim milk**
**1 teaspoon butter or margarine**
**Salt and freshly ground black pepper**

1. Whisk together the eggs and milk.
2. Melt the butter in a nonstick skillet over low heat. Pour the egg mixture into the skillet, and season with salt and pepper.
3. Cook the eggs over low heat, stirring them gently when bubbles begin to rise to the surface and continuing to stir as the eggs set. When they're finished, which takes 4 to 6 minutes, the eggs should be soft but set, with no visible liquid remaining.

NUTRITION PER SERVING

Calories 120 • Fat 9 g • Fiber 0 g • Protein 9 g • Carbohydrates 2 g

# poached eggs

MAKES 2 SERVINGS

Custard dishes are small, round, usually ceramic dishes. You can often find them in grocery stores. For this recipe, however, any small dish that can be immersed in boiling water will do — just make sure that the sides are higher than the water level.

Poached eggs are perfect served on crispy, buttered English muffin halves.

**2 eggs**
**Salt and freshly ground black pepper**

1. Fill a pot with about 2 inches of water and bring to a boil. Lower the heat to medium.
2. Crack an egg into a shallow custard dish. Slip the dish into the pot of boiling water. Don't worry if water spills in over the egg.
3. Simmer for 3 to 5 minutes, or until the egg is done to your satisfaction. Remove the dish from the pot, using tongs, and pat the egg dry with a paper towel if any water has seeped in. Sprinkle with salt and pepper.
4. Repeat steps 2 and 3 for the second egg.

NUTRITION PER SERVING

Calories 70 • Fat 5 g • Fiber 0 g • Protein 6 g • Carbohydrates 0 g

# huevos rancheros

MAKES 2 SERVINGS

This Mexican favorite can be very high in calories, but this version keeps things light with fat-free beans and salsa. Buy a can of fat-free refried beans and keep the leftovers in an airtight container in the refrigerator for three to five days. Use them in burritos, tacos, or quesadillas.

**2 eggs**
**1 teaspoon skim milk**
**2 small flour tortillas**
**½ teaspoon butter**
**3 heaping tablespoons fat-free refried beans**
**Hot sauce**
**Salt and freshly ground black pepper**
**2 tablespoons salsa**
**¼ cup shredded low-fat cheddar cheese (optional)**

1. Beat together the eggs and milk.
2. Place the tortillas directly on the rack in a cold oven. Turn the oven to 300°F and heat the tortillas for approximately 5 minutes, or until warm and slightly crispy.
3. While the tortillas are warming, melt the butter in a small nonstick skillet over medium heat. Add the eggs and stir gently until they are set. Transfer the eggs to a serving plate and place another plate upside down over them to keep them warm.
4. In the same skillet, heat the beans until warmed through.
5. Place the tortillas on fresh plates. Spread beans over the tortillas, top with eggs, sprinkle with hot sauce and salt and pepper to taste, and finish with a spoonful of salsa and a scattering of cheese, if using.

NUTRITION PER SERVING

Calories 200 • Fat 8 g • Fiber 2 g • Protein 10 g • Carbohydrates 21 g

# breakfast burrito

MAKES 1 SERVING

If you have nutritional yeast, add a tablespoon to the scrambled eggs for a healthy boost.

**½ tablespoon butter or vegetable oil**
**Chopped vegetables of choice (onion, pepper, tomato, beans, and so on)**
**2 eggs**
**Salt and freshly ground black pepper**
**1 flour or corn tortilla**
**2 tablespoons shredded cheese (cheddar or Monterey Jack works well)**

1. Melt the butter in a skillet over medium heat. Add the vegetables and sauté until they are just beginning to become tender.

2. While the vegetables are cooking, beat the eggs in a small bowl and season with salt and pepper to taste. Pour the eggs into the pan with the vegetables and cook, stirring occasionally, until they are done to your liking.

3. Place the tortilla on a plate or, for ultimate carry-with-you convenience, a sheet of aluminum foil. Spread the cheese over the middle of the tortilla. Place the egg mixture on top. Fold up the bottom of the tortilla and bring in the sides. If you're using aluminum foil, wrap it around the tortilla to help it to maintain its shape. Enjoy!

NUTRITION PER SERVING

Calories 380 • Fat 20 g • Fiber 2 g • Protein 20 g • Carbohydrates 29 g

# tomato-basil omelets

MAKES 2 SERVINGS

Tomato sauce and basil offer an unexpected twist to this omelet.

**4 eggs**
**2 teaspoons butter**
**2 tablespoons tomato sauce**
**1 teaspoon dried basil**
**Salt and freshly ground black pepper**

1. Crack the eggs into a small bowl and beat them.
2. Melt 1 teaspoon of the butter in a nonstick skillet over medium heat. Add half of the eggs and cook for 1 to 2 minutes, or until the edges begin to pull away from the pan and the middle begins to solidify.
3. Spread 1 tablespoon of the tomato sauce on half of the omelet, sprinkle with half of the basil, then fold over. Season with salt and pepper; serve.
4. Repeat steps 2 and 3 with the remaining ingredients for a second omelet.

NUTRITION PER SERVING
Calories 180 • Fat 13 g • Fiber 0 g • Protein 12 g • Carbohydrates 3 g

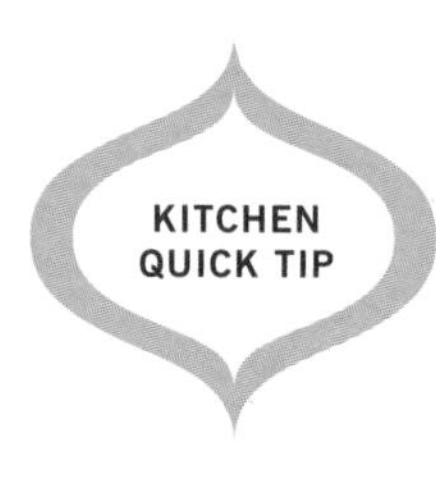


## microwave omelets

Omelets can also be done completely in the microwave. Omit the butter and cook the eggs in a 9-inch pie plate for about 2 minutes on the high setting. If your microwave doesn't have a turntable, rotate the dish every 30 seconds. When the eggs are fully cooked, add your filling ingredients, then fold the eggs over and heat for an additional 20 seconds.

# spicy tomato-corn omelets

MAKES 2 SERVINGS

For those of you who need a kick to wake up in the morning, the hot sauce in this omelet may do the trick. Add another teaspoon if you need serious help. If you don't have a microwave in which to heat the vegetables and hot sauce, don't worry — just don't heat them up.

**½ cup corn kernels**
**1 medium tomato, chopped, or ¼ cup salsa**
**1 teaspoon hot sauce**
**4 eggs**
**¼ cup water**
**2 teaspoons butter**
**¼ cup shredded low-fat cheddar cheese**

1. Combine the corn, tomato, and hot sauce in a small bowl and heat on high in the microwave for 1 minute. Set aside.
2. Beat together the eggs and water in a small bowl.
3. Melt 1 teaspoon of the butter in a nonstick skillet over medium heat. Add half of the eggs and cook for 1 to 2 minutes, or until the edges begin to pull away from the pan and the middle begins to solidify.
4. Remove the skillet from the stovetop and spoon half of the corn-tomato mixture onto half of the omelet. Sprinkle with half of the cheese and fold the eggs over the filling with a spatula. Return to the stovetop for 30 seconds more, then carefully remove the omelet from the pan to a serving plate.
5. Repeat steps 3 and 4 with the remaining ingredients for a second omelet.

**NUTRITION PER SERVING**
Calories 240 • Fat 14 g • Fiber 1 g • Protein 17 g • Carbohydrates 11 g

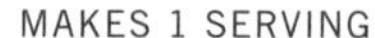

# frittata

MAKES 1 SERVING

You're going to need a pan that can go straight under a broiler for this one — no plastic handles.

**½ teaspoon extra-virgin olive oil**
**2 tablespoons finely chopped onion**
**¼ cup chopped broccoli**
**2 mushrooms, sliced**
**2 eggs**
**1 teaspoon skim milk**
**Pinch of salt**
**Grated Parmesan cheese (optional)**

1. Preheat the broiler.
2. Heat the oil in an ovenproof skillet over medium heat. Add the vegetables and sauté until softened. Transfer the vegetables to a plate and set aside. Don't wash the pan yet.
3. Beat together the eggs, milk, and salt. Pour the egg mixture into the skillet and cook over medium heat just until the bottom begins to solidify. Add the vegetables to the egg mixture, making sure that they are evenly dispersed.
4. Remove the skillet from the stovetop and place it under the broiler for about 5 minutes, or until the frittata's top is firm. Sprinkle with Parmesan, if using, and serve.

NUTRITION PER SERVING

Calories 200 • Fat 12 g • Fiber 2 g • Protein 14 g • Carbohydrates 8 g

# quiche-adilla

MAKES 2 SERVINGS

This recipe is inexpensive and easy to make, uses very few dishes (who doesn't hate to wash up?), and produces a healthy staple that you can keep in the fridge and use throughout the week.

**1–2 tablespoons extra-virgin olive oil**
**3–4 garlic cloves, minced**
**½ medium onion, chopped**
**½ red bell pepper, seeded and chopped (optional)**
**1 (10-ounce) package frozen chopped spinach, thawed and drained**
**1 tomato, chopped**
**Salt**
**Freshly ground black pepper**
**Crushed red pepper flakes**
**2 eggs**
**2 whole-wheat tortillas**
**½ cup shredded mozzarella cheese**

1. Heat the oil in a skillet over medium heat. Add the garlic, onion, and red pepper, if using, and sauté until the onion is translucent.
2. Add the spinach and continue to cook until the spinach is heated through and most of the liquid has evaporated.
3. Add the chopped tomato and cook until most of the moisture has evaporated; season with salt, pepper, and red pepper flakes to taste.
4. Remove all but about 1 cup of the spinach mixture and store in a separate container (for other uses; see below). Crack the eggs into the remaining spinach mixture and scramble.
5. In a separate skillet, heat a drizzle of olive oil. Add 1 tortilla and top with the spinach and egg mixture, a layer of mozzarella, and the other tortilla. Cook until browned on the bottom, then flip and cook until browned on the other side. Serve warm.

**NOTE:** The remaining spinach mixture is a great staple! It can be warmed and served as a delicious side dish or mixed with some cooked ground beef or turkey, marinara sauce, mozzarella cheese, and pasta to make a deconstructed lasagna.

NUTRITION PER SERVING

Calories 375 • Fat 17 g • Fiber 8 g • Protein 18 g • Carbohydrates 38 g

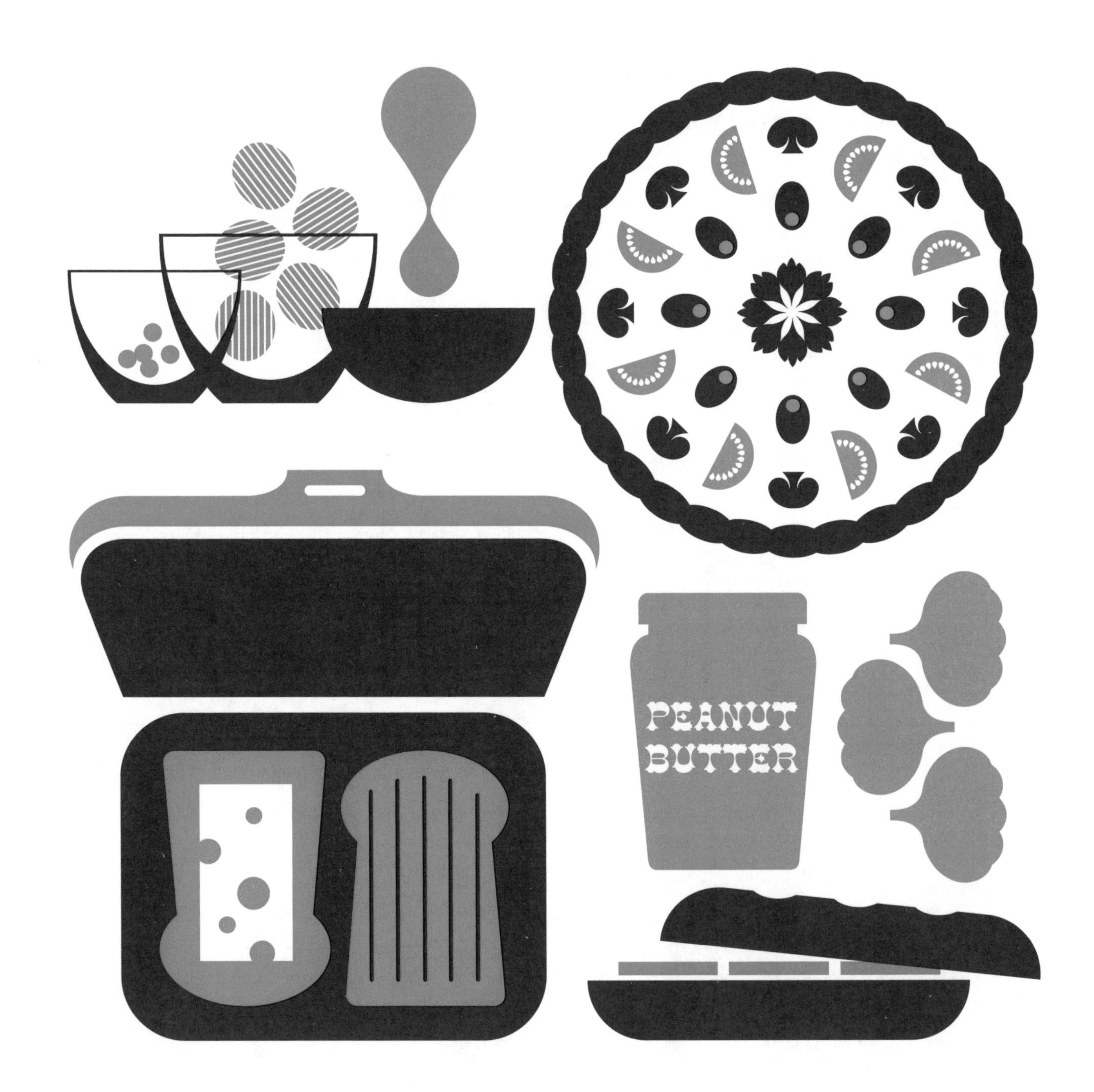
PEANUT
BUTTER

# chapter 3

## appetizers & quick snacks

This section is a great resource if you are having company. Even though the recipes are quick and easy, your guests will think that you've been in the kitchen for days. In addition, many of the appetizers included here are just dressy snacks, so if you are in the mood to munch, this is the chapter for you.

Quick snacks are what you should be nibbling on instead of candy bars, potato chips, or microwave popcorn. Everyone can attest to the formidable nature of that sudden urge to snack. Most of these recipes don't take any longer to prepare than the time it would take you to dash down to a vending machine for a candy bar.

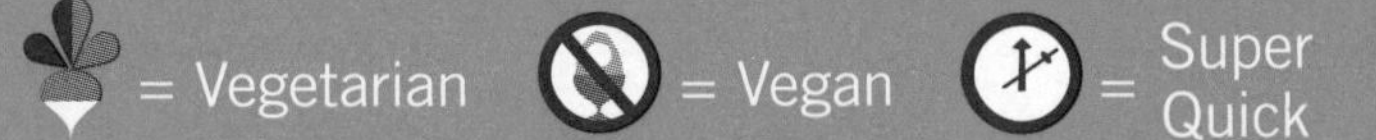 = Vegetarian 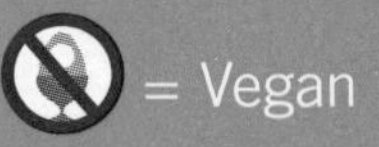 = Vegan 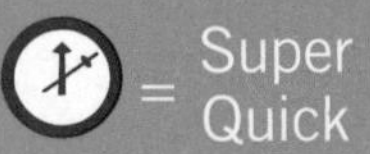 = Super Quick 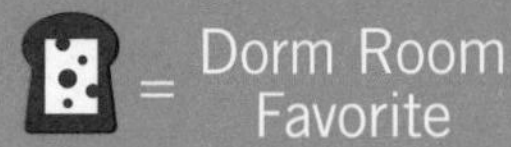 = Dorm Room Favorite

# roasted red pepper and avocado bites

MAKES 8 SERVINGS

This English muffin–based recipe is a satisfying informal snack for any number of people. Plan for a half muffin per person as a between-meals snack or a full muffin with a salad or raw vegetables as a meal.

**4 whole-wheat English muffins**
**½ red onion, chopped**
**1 avocado, pitted, peeled, and sliced**
**1 roasted red pepper (see recipe page 53)**
**1 cup shredded low-fat cheddar cheese**
**¼ cup grated Parmesan cheese**

1. Preheat the broiler.
2. Split the muffins in half, place on a cookie sheet, and toast under the broiler for 2 minutes.
3. Divide the onion among the toasted muffins. Place 1 slice of avocado and 1 large piece of pepper on each muffin half. Spread the cheddar cheese on top of the muffins, and then sprinkle with Parmesan.
4. Broil until the cheese is bubbly and browned, about 2 minutes.

NUTRITION PER SERVING
Calories 150 • Fat 6 g • Fiber 4 g • Protein 8 g • Carbohydrates 17 g

# nachos supreme

MAKES 6 SERVINGS

An all-time favorite on everyone's list. If you have guacamole or sour cream on hand, add a big dollop to the hot nachos. This is easy to make in the microwave as well.

**5 ounces (approximately) baked tortilla chips**
**¼ cup pitted and sliced black olives**
**¼ cup chopped onion**
**½ cup salsa**
**1 cup shredded low-fat cheddar cheese**

1. Preheat the broiler.
2. Spread the chips evenly on a baking sheet. Sprinkle with the olives and onion, then spoon salsa over all. Top with cheese.
3. Broil for about 2 minutes, or until the cheese is melted.

NUTRITION PER SERVING

Calories 140 • Fat 3 g • Fiber 2 g • Protein 7 g • Carbohydrates 24 g

## bulking up

If you'd like to bulk up these nachos, try adding some refried beans, cooked ground beef, chili, chopped tomato, or diced green pepper. You can also try a variety of cheeses. The possibilities are endless.

# south of the border chip dip

MAKES 8 SERVINGS

This one gets a big star. Serve the dip with tortilla chips or a plate of raw vegetables. Celery, broccoli, and bell pepper strips all work well.

- **1 (16-ounce) can fat-free refried beans**
- **1 cup low-fat sour cream**
- **1 tablespoon taco seasoning**
- **1 cup salsa**
- **1 cup shredded low-fat cheddar cheese**
- **1 tomato, diced**
- **¼ cup fresh cilantro leaves (optional)**

1. Spread the beans evenly in a small casserole dish or pie plate to form the bottom layer of the dip.
2. Mix together the sour cream and taco seasoning and spread evenly over the beans. Top with the salsa.
3. Spread the cheese, tomato, and cilantro, if using, evenly over the salsa. Serve at room temperature.

NUTRITION PER SERVING

Calories 120 • Fat 2 g • Fiber 4 g • Protein 9 g • Carbohydrates 17 g

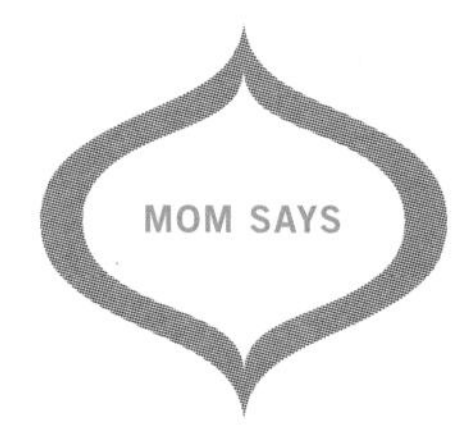


## keeping crackers

In humid weather, keep crackers and chips in an airtight container in the refrigerator to prevent them from turning soft or soggy.

# guacamole

MAKES 6 SERVINGS

Guacamole doesn't keep that well in the refrigerator — it tends to turn brown — so if you're making this recipe for just yourself, halve the ingredients. It's true that more than 80 percent of this recipe's calories come from fat — that's from the avocado. However, the fat in avocados is unsaturated, not the saturated kind that doctors and nutritionists warn against. The fat in avocados is actually good for you.

**2 avocados, pitted and peeled**
**1 tablespoon lemon juice**
**2 tablespoons lime juice**
**1 tablespoon finely chopped onion**
**1 teaspoon salt**
**½ teaspoon chili powder**
**Cayenne pepper to taste**
**1 ripe jalapeño pepper, finely chopped (to reduce the heat, remove the seeds)**
**1 ripe tomato, chopped (optional)**
**Corn chips for serving**

1. Mash the avocados with a fork in a small bowl. If you like your guacamole extra smooth, purée the avocado flesh in a blender or food processor.

2. Add the lemon and lime juice, the onion, salt, chili powder, cayenne, jalapeño, and tomato, if using, and mix well. Serve immediately with corn chips.

NUTRITION PER SERVING

Calories 110 • Fat 10 g • Fiber 5 g • Protein 1 g • Carbohydrates 7 g

# spicy edamame snacks

  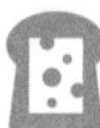

MAKES 4 SERVINGS

Edamame is another name for green soybeans. These tasty beans are low in fat and calories but rich in protein and fiber, and they are incredibly delicious.

**1 (10-ounce) bag frozen, shelled edamame beans**
**1 tablespoon chile oil (sesame oil infused with red chiles)**
**2 tablespoons low-sodium soy sauce**

1. Place the edamame beans in a microwave-safe dish with a lid. Add the chile oil and soy sauce to the beans. Place the lid on the container and shake to coat all the beans with the sauce.
2. Open 1 corner of the lid as a vent. Place the container in the microwave and heat until all of the beans are thawed and not raw to the taste (about 3 minutes, though you will have to experiment with the timing). Eat hot or cold.

NUTRITION PER SERVING

Calories 120 • Fat 7 g • Fiber 4 g • Protein 8 g • Carbohydrates 8 g

# deviled eggs

MAKES 6 SERVINGS

Refrigerate any leftovers, and be sure to eat them within three days of preparation.

**6 hard-boiled eggs, peeled and halved lengthwise (see page 31)**
**3 tablespoons nonfat plain yogurt**
**1 tablespoon diced celery**
**Salt and freshly ground black pepper**
**Curry powder**

1. Scoop the yolks out of the eggs.
2. Blend the yogurt, celery, and a pinch of salt with the yolks in a small bowl. Overfill each egg-white half with the yolk mixture.
3. Sprinkle with salt, pepper, and curry powder to taste. Refrigerate before serving.

NUTRITION PER SERVING
Calories 80 • Fat 5 g • Fiber 0 g • Protein 7 g • Carbohydrates 1 g

# ants on a log

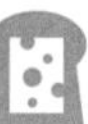

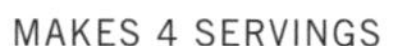

MAKES 4 SERVINGS

It seems that the older we get, the more we appreciate our childhood classics.

**4 celery stalks, trimmed and cleaned**
**1½ tablespoons peanut butter**
**Raisins**

1. Cut the celery into finger-length pieces. (Don't split the stalks lengthwise — you'll need the trough in the center.)
2. Fill the trough of each piece with peanut butter, and top with raisins.

NUTRITION PER SERVING
Calories 170 • Fat 3.5 g • Fiber 3 g • Protein 3 g • Carbohydrates 37 g

## powered-up crispy treats

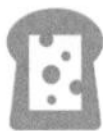

MAKES 6 TO 8 SERVINGS

Easy, delicious, and cheap!

**1 cup peanut butter (smooth or crunchy)**
**1 cup orange juice**
**1 cup dried fruit (raisins, apricots, bananas, apples, cranberries, or a mix of all)**
**2 cups puffed rice cereal**

Stir together all ingredients with a wooden spoon in a large bowl. Shape into walnut-size balls. Store in the refrigerator in snack bags ready to grab and go!

NUTRITION PER SERVING
Calories 380 • Fat 22 g • Fiber 4 g • Protein 12 g • Carbohydrates 38 g

## cereal balls to go

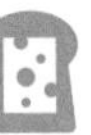

MAKES 4 SERVINGS

These easy-to-make snacks allow you to take breakfast with you when you're in a hurry.

**2 cups crushed whole-grain cereal flakes (such as Wheaties)**
**6 tablespoons honey**
**½ cup peanut butter (smooth or crunchy)**
**½ cup nonfat dry milk powder**

Stir together all ingredients with a wooden spoon in a large bowl. Shape into walnut-size balls. Store in the refrigerator in snack bags ready to grab and go!

NUTRITION PER SERVING
Calories 390 • Fat 17 g • Fiber 3 g • Protein 15 g • Carbohydrates 52 g

# crab-stuffed mushrooms

MAKES 6 SERVINGS

Very easy to make yet also very delicious. If you have leftover stuffing mixture, mix it with a little sour cream and serve it as a dip for crackers, chips, or vegetables.

**Cooking spray**
**24 medium mushrooms**
**1 (8-ounce) package cream cheese, softened**
**1 cup cooked and flaked crab (drained canned is fine)**
**¼ teaspoon garlic powder**
**¼ teaspoon dried basil**
**1 teaspoon lemon juice**
**2 dashes Worcestershire sauce**
**2 scallions, thinly sliced**
**¼ teaspoon lemon-pepper seasoning**
**½ cup shredded cheddar cheese**
**2 tablespoons grated Parmesan cheese**

1. Lightly grease a large baking dish with cooking spray.
2. Clean the mushrooms, brushing or wiping off any dirt with a damp cloth. Remove the stems, setting the caps aside. Discard half of the mushroom stems. Trim the tough bottoms from the remaining stems and finely chop.
3. Combine the chopped mushroom stems, cream cheese, crab, garlic powder, basil, lemon juice, Worcestershire, scallions, and lemon-pepper seasoning in a large bowl, mixing thoroughly.
4. Fill the mushroom caps with the cream cheese mixture. Set the caps in the prepared baking dish, stuffing side up. Sprinkle the cheeses over the stuffed caps. Refrigerate for at least 4 hours (overnight is fine).
5. Preheat oven to 450°F. Bake mushrooms for 15 to 20 minutes, until the caps are hot and the cheese is bubbly and browned.

NUTRITION PER SERVING

Calories 190 • Fat 15 g • Fiber 1 g • Protein 12 g • Carbohydrates 4 g

# mushrooms parmesan

MAKES 3 SERVINGS

When you remove the stems from the mushroom caps, make sure that you get the whole stem, and that you're not just cracking the top off. There should be plenty of room in the caps for stuffing.

**9 medium mushrooms**
**1 tablespoon butter**
**Grated Parmesan cheese**
**Salt and freshly ground black pepper**

1. Preheat the broiler.
2. Wipe the mushrooms clean with a damp cloth. Pull the stems out of the mushroom caps. Place the caps upside down on a foil-lined cookie sheet.
3. Trim and dice the mushroom stems and stuff them back into the caps. Place a sliver of butter in each cap, and sprinkle Parmesan, salt, and pepper over each.
4. Broil for approximately 3 minutes, or until the mushrooms are light brown.

NUTRITION PER SERVING

Calories 50 • Fat 4.5 g • Fiber 1 g • Protein 2 g • Carbohydrates 2 g

# italian mushrooms

MAKES 4 SERVINGS

Keep napkins handy when you serve this tasty but messy appetizer.

**12 bite-size mushrooms**
**1½ cups Italian dressing (see page 115 for our own recipe)**
**1 tablespoon grated Parmesan cheese**

1. Wipe the mushrooms clean with a damp cloth and trim the stems.
2. Place the mushrooms in a bowl and cover with the dressing. Add the Parmesan and stir well. Refrigerate for 2 hours.
3. Drain the dressing from the mushrooms, and serve with toothpicks.

NUTRITION PER SERVING
Calories 270 • Fat 25 g • Fiber 0 g • Protein 2 g • Carbohydrates 10 g

# mustard-horseradish vegetable dip

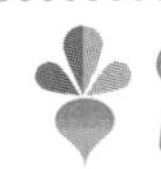
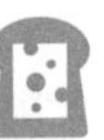

MAKES 6 SERVINGS

Cut up various vegetables — carrots, broccoli, cauliflower, celery, and radishes — and serve beside the dip. It's great for gatherings.

**4½ tablespoons nonfat plain yogurt**
**5 teaspoons Dijon mustard**
**3 tablespoons horseradish**

Combine all ingredients and mix well. Serve immediately.

NUTRITION PER SERVING
Calories 10 • Fat 0 g • Fiber 0 g • Protein 1 g • Carbohydrates 2 g

# artichoke dip

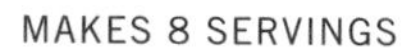

MAKES 8 SERVINGS

This classic dip is traditionally high in calories, but a few simple substitutions cut the fat and boost the health benefits. Add a selection of raw vegetables for dipping and this becomes a very healthy treat.

**1 (15-ounce) can artichoke hearts in water, drained**
**¼ cup low-fat mayonnaise**
**¼ cup nonfat plain yogurt**
**½ cup grated Parmesan cheese**
**¼ teaspoon freshly ground black pepper**
**1 teaspoon chopped fresh parsley (optional)**
**Crackers or a sliced baguette**

1. Preheat the oven to 400°F.
2. Coarsely chop the artichoke hearts. Combine the artichoke hearts with the mayonnaise, yogurt, Parmesan, and pepper; mix thoroughly. Spread evenly in a small casserole dish or loaf pan.
3. Bake for 20 minutes, or until hot and lightly browned. Remove from the oven, top with parsley, if using, and serve with crackers or sliced French bread rounds.

NUTRITION PER SERVING
Calories 60 • Fat 2 g • Fiber 5 g • Protein 4 g • Carbohydrates 8 g

# baked garlic

MAKES 6 SERVINGS

Soft, spreadable baked garlic is wonderful on sandwiches or as a topping for vegetables.

**1 whole bulb garlic**

1. Preheat the oven to 400°F.
2. Remove any loose, papery outer leaves of the garlic bulb. Cut off the stem end of the bulb so that each clove is open at the top.
3. Set the bulb in a pan or on a baking sheet and bake for 45 minutes. Garlic is finished when the cloves are tender and the husks are golden brown.

NUTRITION PER SERVING

Calories 5 • Fat 0 g • Fiber 0 g • Protein 0 g • Carbohydrates 2 g

# roasted red pepper

MAKES 2 SERVINGS

Roasted red peppers are most commonly enjoyed in sandwiches or on salads.

**1 red bell pepper**

1. Preheat the oven to 350°F.
2. Line a baking sheet with aluminum foil. Place the whole pepper on the pan and bake for 30 minutes, turning occasionally.
3. Remove the pepper from the oven, place it in a ziplock bag, and seal the bag. When the pepper is cool enough to handle, remove it from the bag and peel off its skin. Cut the pepper open and remove the seeds, then slice the flesh into long strips.

NUTRITION PER SERVING

Calories 25 • Fat 0 g • Fiber 2 g • Protein 1 g • Carbohydrates 5 g

# gourmet endive

MAKES 8 SERVINGS

Simple, elegant, and delicious, this appealing finger food goes fast at get-togethers.

**5 tablespoons reduced-fat cream cheese**
**1 tablespoon dried oregano**
**1 teaspoon dried basil**
**¼ teaspoon salt**
**¼ teaspoon freshly ground black pepper**
**3 Belgian endives**

1. Combine the cream cheese with the oregano, basil, salt, and pepper in a small bowl and mix thoroughly.
2. Slice off the roots of the endives and separate the leaves. Arrange the leaves on a plate. Spread the cream cheese into the troughs and serve.

NUTRITION PER SERVING
Calories 25 • Fat 1.5 g • Fiber 1 g • Protein 1 g • Carbohydrates 2 g

# vegetable cream cheese

 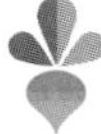 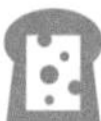

MAKES 8 SERVINGS

Refrigerate and use as a topping for bagels or as a spread in sandwiches or roll-ups.

**1 (8-ounce) container nonfat cream cheese**
**1 scallion, sliced**
**1 teaspoon finely diced carrot**
**1 teaspoon finely diced green or red bell pepper**

Combine all ingredients in a bowl and mix thoroughly. Store in the refrigerator.

NUTRITION PER SERVING
Calories 30 • Fat 0 g • Fiber 0 g • Protein 4 g • Carbohydrates 2 g

# honey butter

MAKES 6 SERVINGS

This is a great spread to serve over toast, English muffins, or pancakes — the extra flavor allows you to use it in moderation.

**2 tablespoons butter**
**2 tablespoons honey**
**1 teaspoon vanilla**

Melt the butter in a small saucepan over medium heat. Add the honey and vanilla, and mix well. Use immediately or refrigerate for later.

NUTRITION PER SERVING
Calories 60 • Fat 4 g • Fiber 0 g • Protein 0 g • Carbohydrates 6 g

# ricotta crostini

MAKES 1 SERVING

This snack tastes best when the bread is grilled, but you can make it with a slice of toast. Drizzle the oil over the bread after it comes out of the toaster.

**1 thick slice of crusty, good bread, such as ciabatta**
**2 teaspoons extra-virgin olive oil**
**2 tablespoons ricotta cheese**
**1 teaspoon lemon zest**
**honey**

1. Drizzle bread with olive oil.
2. Grill or broil both sides of the bread on medium heat until you have obvious grill marks and the crusts are a bit charred, about 4 minutes.
3. Spread the cheese on the bread, grate the lemon zest over the cheese, and drizzle a little honey over the entire thing. Eat immediately.

NUTRITION PER SERVING
Calories 430 • Fat 14 g • Fiber 3 g • Protein 15 g • Carbohydrates 62 g

# your basic hummus

MAKES 10 SERVINGS

Great for sandwiches, bagels, and dipping, hummus is an all-purpose food. You'll need a food processor to make it.

**1 (15-ounce) can chickpeas (also known as garbanzo beans)**
**2 garlic cloves, minced**
**¼ cup sesame tahini**
**⅓ cup lemon juice**
**¼ teaspoon cayenne pepper**

1. Drain the chickpeas, saving the liquid. Put the beans into the bowl of a food processor.
2. Add the garlic, tahini, lemon juice, and cayenne and blend until smooth. If the mixture is too thick add some of the liquid from the beans.

NUTRITION PER SERVING
Calories 200 • Fat 6 g • Fiber 8 g • Protein 10 g • Carbohydrates 27 g

## what is tahini?

Tahini is a Middle Eastern paste made of ground sesame seeds. You will find it in the ethnic food section of your supermarket.

# lower-fat hummus

MAKES 12 SERVINGS

Hummus is full of protein but it often contains a lot of fat. This is a satisfying lower-fat alternative.

**1 (15-ounce) can chickpeas, rinsed and drained**
**1–2 tablespoons peanut butter**
**2 garlic cloves, minced**
**2 tablespoons extra-virgin olive oil**
**2 tablespoons lemon juice**
**¼ cup nonfat plain yogurt**
**1 teaspoon salt**
**1 teaspoon freshly ground black pepper**
**Chopped olives, peppers, parsley, or anything else you might like**

1. Combine the chickpeas and peanut butter in the bowl of a food processor and blend until smooth. Add the garlic, olive oil, and lemon juice and blend again.
2. Pulse in dollops of the yogurt until the mixture reaches your preferred consistency. Add salt and pepper to taste, as well as any other extras you might like. Refrigerate for at least 1 hour before serving.

NUTRITION PER SERVING

Calories 160 • Fat 5 g • Fiber 6 g • Protein 7 g • Carbohydrates 23 g

# b. l. t. tater

MAKES 1 SERVING

It's warm, filling, easy to make, inexpensive, and yummy!

**1 medium baking potato**
**1 cup chopped lettuce**
**2 tablespoons cooked, crumbled bacon, or artificial bacon bits**
**2 tablespoons chopped tomato**
**2 tablespoons salad dressing of your choice (nonfat or low-fat)**

1. Pierce the raw potato several times with the tines of a fork. Place the potato on a microwave-safe plate. Microwave on the high setting until tender, 8 to 10 minutes.
2. Arrange the lettuce on a plate. Place the potato on top of the lettuce and cut it open with a knife, spreading it over the lettuce.
3. Top the potato with bacon pieces, chopped tomato, and the dressing of your choice. Serve immediately.

NUTRITION PER SERVING

Calories 260 • Fat 5 g • Fiber 5 g • Protein 14 g • Carbohydrates 41 g

# quesadillas

MAKES 4 SERVINGS

Everyone loves warm, melted cheese. Invent your own quesadillas with any ingredients you enjoy with cheese.

**¾ cup shredded low-fat cheddar cheese**
**½ tomato, diced**
**2 medium mushrooms, cleaned and diced**
**¼ medium onion, diced**
**4 flour tortillas**

1. Preheat the oven to 350°F.
2. Combine the cheese, tomato, mushrooms, and onion in a small bowl.
3. Place the tortillas on a baking sheet. Spread one-fourth of the cheese mixture over half of each tortilla.
4. Bake for 6 to 8 minutes, or until the cheese is bubbling. Remove from the oven. Fold the bare half of each tortilla over the filled half. Serve warm.

NUTRITION PER SERVING
Calories 200 • Fat 5 g • Fiber 2 g • Protein 10 g • Carbohydrates 27 g

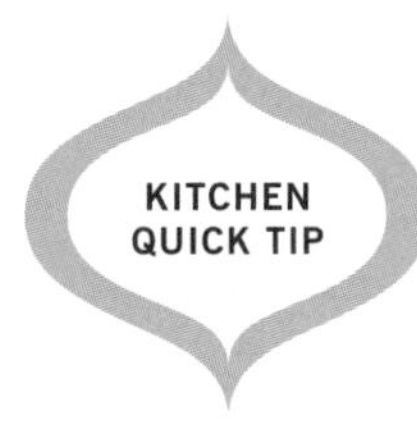


## 6 quick fillings for a tortilla

- Fat-free refried beans, tomato, and cheese
- Black beans, corn, and cinnamon
- Grilled or sautéed vegetables — onions, peppers, zucchini, eggplant, or whatever's lingering in the refrigerator — with nonfat sour cream
- Cottage cheese and salsa
- Tomato, avocado, and lemon or lime juice
- Leftover chicken or beef, salsa, and nonfat sour cream

# open-face quesadillas

MAKES 2 SERVINGS

The simplest, best-tasting quesadillas ever — and they're low-fat.

**1 large tortilla**
**4 tablespoons chile con queso (found in the snack aisle with the dips)**
**¼ cup chopped green bell pepper**
**¼ cup chopped tomato**
**¼ cup chopped onion**
**½ cup shredded low-fat cheddar cheese**

1. Preheat the broiler.
2. Heat the tortilla in a skillet over low heat until it is lightly toasted.
3. Place the tortilla on a baking sheet. Spread the chile con queso over the tortilla, leaving a bit of bare crust around the outside like a pizza. Scatter the vegetables over the top of the tortilla. Top with the cheese. Broil for 3 to 5 minutes, or until the cheese is completely melted and bubbly.
4. Slice the quesadilla into 6 pieces (a pizza cutter works well for this), and enjoy immediately.

NUTRITION PER SERVING
Calories 190 • Fat 7 g • Fiber 2 g • Protein 10 g • Carbohydrates 20 g

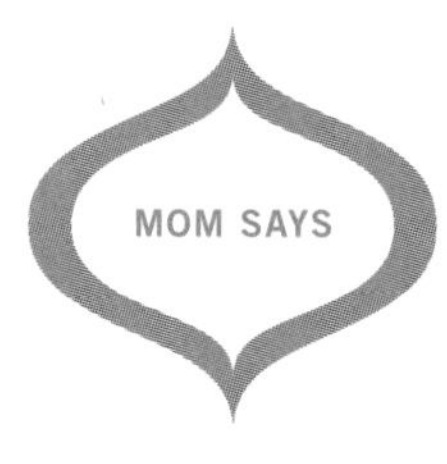


## quesadillas on the (indoor) grill

Your George Foreman Grill is great for making quesadillas. The filling heats up quickly and evenly and you won't have to flip the quesadilla. Coat both the top and bottom grills with a quick spritz of cooking spray to prevent the tortillas from sticking. Don't use your George Foreman for an open-face quesadilla, though.

# chicken & bacon quesadillas

MAKES 8 TO 10 SERVINGS

Everyone loves this snack! You can make a batch of the filling ahead of time and keep it in your fridge so that you can enjoy fresh quesadillas all week. If you want to avoid the fat of the bacon, substitute cooked beans — pinto beans or black beans work well.

- **1½ cups shredded cheddar cheese**
- **1 cup chopped cooked chicken (canned is fine)**
- **¾ cup chopped tomatoes**
- **½ cup chopped cooked bacon**
- **½ cup chopped red onion**
- **⅓ cup chopped green chiles (canned is fine)**
- **5 large flour tortillas**
- **Cooking spray**

1. Combine all ingredients except the tortillas and cooking spray in a large bowl. Divide the mixture among the tortillas, spreading it on half of each tortilla. Fold the tortillas in half.
2. Coat a large skillet with cooking spray and heat over medium heat. One by one, place the tortillas in the skillet and cook each side until they are golden brown and the cheese is melted. Recoat the pan as necessary.
3. Cut each tortilla into quarters for serving.

NUTRITION PER SERVING

Calories 230 • Fat 13 g • Fiber 1 g • Protein 14 g • Carbohydrates 15 g

## english muffin pizza

MAKES 1 SERVING

**2 tablespoons tomato sauce**
**1 English muffin, split in half**
**Dried oregano**
**¼ cup shredded low-fat mozzarella cheese**
**2 black olives, pitted and sliced**

1. Preheat the oven to 350°F.
2. Spread the tomato sauce evenly over the English muffin halves. Sprinkle with oregano to taste and the cheese. Top with the olives. Place on a baking sheet and bake for 5 minutes, or until the cheese is melted.

NUTRITION PER SERVING
Calories 230 • Fat 7 g • Fiber 2 g • Protein 13 g • Carbohydrates 30 g

## onion pizza

MAKES 1 SERVING

**1 tablespoon tomato sauce**
**1 small ready-made pizza crust**
**1 slice red onion, chopped**
**¼ cup shredded low-fat mozzarella cheese**

1. Preheat the broiler.
2. Spread the tomato sauce over the pizza crust. Sprinkle with the onion and cover with the cheese, spreading evenly.
3. Broil for about 2 minutes, or until the cheese is melted.

NUTRITION PER SERVING
Calories 260 • Fat 8 g • Fiber 2 g • Protein 13 g • Carbohydrates 37 g

# mushroom pizzas

MAKES 2 SERVINGS

This is a great healthy meal that's full of protein. If you can't find prepackaged bruschetta mix, chop a couple of tomatoes and season them with basil, parsley, and garlic.

**2 large portobello mushrooms**
**1 cup shredded mozzarella cheese**
**1 cup shredded Parmesan cheese**
**Crushed red pepper flakes**
**1 (8-ounce) can cannellini beans, rinsed and drained**
**1 (6- to 10-ounce) container bruschetta mix (the exact size doesn't matter)**

1. Preheat the oven to 350°F.
2. Remove the stems from the mushrooms. Scrape the gills with a spoon to hollow the caps a bit.
3. Mix the cheeses with red pepper flakes to taste. Set half of the cheese mixture aside. Mix the remaining cheese mixture with the beans and bruschetta.
4. Top the 2 mushroom caps with the bruschetta mixture. Sprinkle the remaining cheese on top. Bake for 20 minutes, or until the caps are heated through and the cheese is melted. Serve warm.

NUTRITION PER SERVING

Calories 580 • Fat 35 g • Fiber 7 g • Protein 38 g • Carbohydrates 27 g

# toaster-oven pita pizza

MAKES 1 SERVING

If you're chopping vegetables for another recipe, set some aside in a plastic container in the refrigerator, and you'll be all set to make this quick and easy recipe for lunch the next day!

**1 whole-wheat pita**
**¼ cup tomato sauce**
**Handful of shredded mozzarella (or any type cheese you like)**
**Toppings of your choice (vegetables, pepperoni slices, and so on)**

1. Preheat the broiler of your toaster oven.
2. Place the pita on a toaster broiler pan. Spread the sauce on top of the pita. Sprinkle with cheese and add the toppings. Place in the toaster and broil until the cheese is melted. Eat hot.

NUTRITION PER SERVING
Calories 170 • Fat 6 g • Fiber 3 g • Protein 11 g • Carbohydrates 20 g

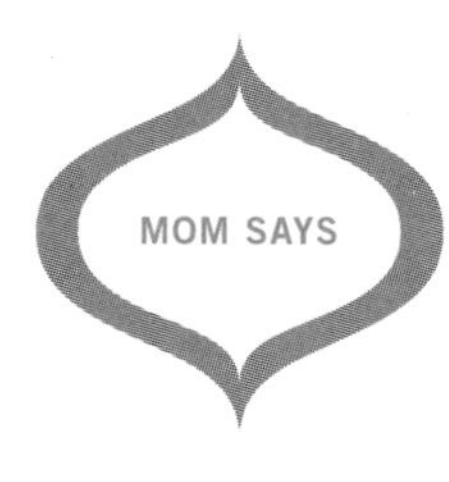


## storing cheese

When returning an opened package of cheese to the refrigerator, remove the original wrapping and place the cheese in an airtight plastic bag. It may seem wasteful to use so much plastic, but you can always recycle the bags, and they will keep your cheese from getting stale and hard.

## grilled cheese and tomato

MAKES 1 SERVING

A classic. Best served with tomato soup.

**1 slice low-fat cheddar cheese**
**2 slices whole-wheat bread**
**1 slice tomato**
**Dried basil**
**1 teaspoon butter**

1. Lay the cheese on 1 slice of bread. Top with the tomato, a pinch of basil, and the second slice of bread.
2. Melt the butter in a small skillet over medium-high heat. Cook the sandwich for about 2 minutes per side, or until the cheese is melted and the bread is golden brown.

NUTRITION PER SERVING
Calories 230 • Fat 13 g • Fiber 4 g • Protein 13 g • Carbohydrates 21 g

## tomato and pesto sandwich

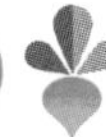

MAKES 1 SERVING

This one is terrific, especially if you have a little pesto left over from last night's dinner. If you don't have homemade pesto, the sandwich will still be delicious with a swipe of store-bought pesto.

**2 slices whole-grain bread**
**½ tablespoon pesto (see page 182, step 1)**
**2 slices tomato**

Toast the bread. Spread the pesto on 1 side of 1 slice of toast. Top with the tomato and the second slice of toast. Serve.

NUTRITION PER SERVING
Calories 180 • Fat 6 g • Fiber 4 g • Protein 9 g • Carbohydrates 24 g

# mozzarella grilled cheese with tomato and arugula

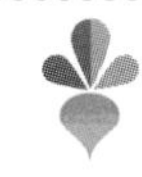

MAKES 1 SERVING

This is a dressed-up version of the traditional grilled cheese sandwich.

- **2 slices ciabatta bread**
- **Extra-virgin olive oil**
- **2 slices mozzarella (smoked mozzarella is especially good)**
- **2 slices low-fat cheddar cheese**
- **2 thin slices tomato**
- **2–3 large arugula leaves**
- **Salt and freshly ground pepper**

1. Heat a skillet over medium heat.
2. Brush 1 side of each slice of bread with olive oil. Place 1 slice of bread oil side down in the hot skillet. Top the bread with mozzarella, cheddar, and then alternating slices of tomato and arugula. Season the tomatoes with salt and pepper as you go. Finish the stack with a final slice of mozzarella and cheddar and the other slice of bread, oil side up.
3. Cook for 2 to 4 minutes, until the bottom slice is golden brown. Then flip the sandwich over and cook the other side. When both sides are golden brown, remove the sandwich from the skillet, cut in half, and enjoy!

NUTRITION PER SERVING

Calories 410 • Fat 27 g • Fiber 2 g • Protein 18 g • Carbohydrates 23 g

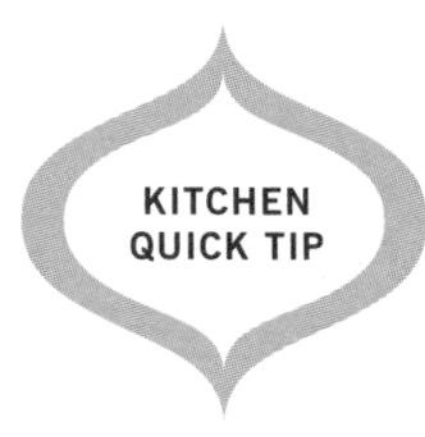


## grilled cheese on your indoor grill

You can make any grilled cheese sandwich on a George Foreman Grill. Assemble the sandwich outside the grill, and cook for 2 to 4 minutes, until both the top and bottom of the sandwich are golden brown. Experiment with all of your favorite toasted sandwiches.

# grilled ham and roast beef sandwich

MAKES 1 SERVING

This sandwich is filling and extremely tasty — as good as anything you'll eat in a deli.

**1 tablespoon butter**
**3 white mushrooms, wiped clean and thinly sliced**
**1 thin slice red onion, separated into rings**
**3 slices ham**
**3 slices roast beef**
**2 slices whole-grain bread**
**1 slice Swiss or cheddar cheese**

1. Melt the butter in a skillet over medium heat. Add the mushrooms and onions to the skillet and sauté 2 to 4 minutes, or until tender.
2. Remove the onions and mushrooms from the skillet and set aside. Add the ham and roast beef to the skillet and cook, stirring often, until sizzling hot. Turn the heat down to low and pour the vegetables back into the skillet with the ham and roast beef to keep warm.
3. Toast the bread.
4. Make a sandwich of the meats and vegetables, topped with the cheese. Grill the sandwich in the skillet until both sides are golden brown and crispy and the cheese is melted. Enjoy!

NUTRITION PER SERVING

Calories 540 • Fat 28 g • Fiber 5 g • Protein 44 g • Carbohydrates 31 g

## hummus sandwich

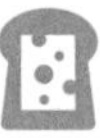

MAKES 1 SERVING

This sandwich is delicious with homemade hummus, but it will still be very tasty if you use your favorite prepared version.

**2 heaping tablespoons hummus (see pages 56 and 57)**
**½ pita pocket**
**4 slices cucumber**
**Handful of bean sprouts**
**Chopped vegetables of your choice — try green or red bell pepper, carrots, or red onion**

Spread the hummus in the pita pocket. Slide in the cucumber slices, sprouts, and any other vegetables that appeal to you.

NUTRITION PER SERVING
Calories 150 • Fat 4 g • Fiber 6 g • Protein 7 g • Carbohydrates 25 g

## tuna melt

MAKES 4 SERVINGS

**2 English muffins, split in half**
**1 (6-ounce) can water-packed tuna, drained**
**1½ tablespoons low-fat mayonnaise**
**Salt and freshly ground black pepper**
**¼ cup shredded low-fat cheddar cheese**

1. Preheat the oven to 350°F. Toast the muffins.
2. Mix the tuna, mayonnaise, and salt and pepper to taste. Place one-quarter of the mixture on each English muffin half. Press with a fork to flatten. Sprinkle the cheese evenly over the tops.
3. Bake until the cheese is melted, about 5 minutes.

NUTRITION PER SERVING
Calories 150 • Fat 4 g • Fiber 1 g • Protein 14 g • Carbohydrates 14 g

# tuna salad wrap

MAKES 1 SERVING

It's easy, quick, and delicious! If you have them, shredded lettuce and diced tomato are great additions to this wrap. The relish may seem like an odd addition but it's delicious. Give it a try!

You can also make the tuna salad with a regular 6-ounce can of tuna in water — just double the remaining ingredients, mix in a separate bowl instead of the tuna container, and season with salt and pepper. The 6-ounce can of tuna will yield 2 servings.

**1 (2.8-ounce) ready-to-eat tuna cup**
**1 teaspoon fat-free or low-fat mayonnaise**
**1 teaspoon mustard**
**1 teaspoon relish (optional)**
**1 small whole-wheat tortilla**

1. Open the tuna cup and add mayonnaise, mustard, and relish, if using, to the tuna. Mix well.
2. Spread the tuna mixture on the tortilla, roll up, and eat.

NUTRITION PER SERVING

Calories 250 • Fat 3 g • Fiber 2 g • Protein 23 g • Carbohydrates 23 g

# pesto turkey sandwich

MAKES 1 SERVING

This recipe packs whole grains, protein, fruit, and vegetables into one amazing sandwich. Skip the mayonnaise and use more pesto if you're a pesto lover.

**2 slices whole-grain bread**
**½ teaspoon mustard**
**1 teaspoon honey**
**1 teaspoon mayonnaise**
**½ teaspoon pesto (see page 182, step 1)**
**3 thin slices apple**
**3 slices turkey**
**1 small tomato, sliced**
**A small handful of sprouts**

1. Toast the bread.
2. Spread the mustard and honey on 1 slice of toast. Spread the mayonnaise and pesto on the other slice of toast. Top 1 slice of toast with the apple, turkey, tomato, sprouts, and the remaining slice of toast. Cut the sandwich in half and enjoy.

NUTRITION PER SERVING

Calories 270 • Fat 5 g • Fiber 6 g • Protein 19 g • Carbohydrates 40 g

# easy chicken philly

MAKES 4 TO 6 SERVINGS

It's easy, delicious, and cheap! This sandwich is a great way to use up leftover chicken.

**2–3 tablespoons butter**
**½ bell pepper (any color), sliced**
**½ red onion, sliced**
**1 loaf soft French bread**
**2–3 ounces cream cheese**
**A few ounces of cooked, sliced chicken**
**A few slices of cheese (any kind)**

1. Melt 1 tablespoon of the butter in a skillet over medium-high heat. Add the pepper and onion slices and sauté until tender. Set aside.
2. Slice the French bread in half lengthwise and spread the remaining butter on its open faces. Place the 2 halves facedown in the skillet to toast. Slice the bread in half crosswise and roast in 2 batches if your skillet is not big enough for the whole loaf.
3. Place one half of the French bread faceup on a microwave-safe plate. Spread the cream cheese over it and top with the peppers and onions, chicken, cheese, and remaining half of the bread.
4. Place the sandwich in a microwave and heat until the cheese is melted, 30 to 45 seconds. Slice and enjoy!

NUTRITION PER SERVING

Calories 180 • Fat 13 g • Fiber 0 g • Protein 8 g • Carbohydrates 7 g

## open-face avocado sandwich

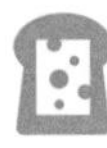

MAKES 2 SERVINGS

Avocado is not a low-fat food, but most of the fat it contains is unsaturated, and it is an excellent source of other nutrients, such as fiber, potassium, B vitamins, and antioxidants.

**2 slices whole-grain sourdough bread**
**1 avocado, pitted, peeled, and sliced**
**Salt and freshly ground black pepper**
**½ lime, cut in half**
**Fresh cilantro leaves**

Lay the bread on plates. Arrange the avocado slices over the 2 slices of bread. Sprinkle with a pinch of salt and plenty of fresh pepper. Squeeze the juice from one-quarter of a lime over each slice. Use a fork to press the avocado into the bread. Arrange a handful of cilantro leaves on top. Enjoy.

NUTRITION PER SERVING
Calories 260 • Fat 16 g • Fiber 9 g • Protein 5 g • Carbohydrates 25 g

## cottage cheese on a bagel

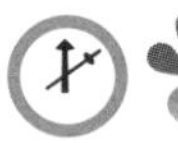

MAKES 1 SERVING

**½ bagel**
**2 tablespoons fat-free cottage cheese**
**Cinnamon and sugar**

1. Toast the bagel.
2. Top the toasted bagel with cottage cheese; sprinkle with cinnamon and sugar to taste. Enjoy.

NUTRITION PER SERVING
Calories 120 • Fat 0.5 g • Fiber 1 g • Protein 7 g • Carbohydrates 22 g

# the chagel

MAKES 1 SERVING

Substitute a fried egg if you prefer fried to scrambled. If you don't have a microwave, you can melt the cheese in a broiler — remember to preheat it.

**Cooking spray**
**1 egg, beaten**
**1 bagel of choice**
**1 tablespoon shredded low-fat mozzarella cheese**
**Salt and freshly ground black pepper**
**Cayenne pepper**

1. Coat a nonstick skillet with cooking spray and heat over medium heat. Add the egg and cook, stirring gently, until firm and dry.
2. While the egg is cooking, slice and toast the bagel.
3. Spoon the egg onto 1 bagel half. Sprinkle the cheese on top and heat in the microwave (or broil) until the cheese is melted. Season with salt, pepper, and cayenne to taste. Top with the other bagel half and enjoy.

NUTRITION PER SERVING

Calories 280 • Fat 7 g • Fiber 2 g • Protein 15 g • Carbohydrates 38 g

# quick western sandwich

MAKES 1 SERVING

This is a classic sandwich that's delicious as a snack or as a light meal with a salad.

**½ teaspoon butter**
**1 egg, beaten**
**1 scallion, sliced**
**1 tablespoon shredded low-fat mozzarella cheese**
**1 teaspoon hot sauce (optional)**
**2 slices whole-wheat bread**
**1 slice ham**

1. Melt the butter in a medium skillet over medium-high heat. Add the egg, scallion, cheese, and hot sauce, if desired. Cook, stirring gently, for 2 to 3 minutes, or until firm and dry.
2. While the egg mixture cooks, toast the 2 slices of bread.
3. Place the egg and onion mixture on 1 slice of toast. Top with the ham and the second slice of toast. Cut the sandwich in 2 and serve immediately.

NUTRITION PER SERVING

Calories 210 • Fat 10 g • Fiber 4 g • Protein 16 g • Carbohydrates 22 g

# green egg sandwich

MAKES 1 SERVING

This hot and tasty sandwich makes a great meal any time of the day. It goes very well with fresh fruit!

**1 teaspoon extra-virgin olive oil**
**2 eggs**
**2 slices whole-grain bread**
**2 tablespoons hummus**
**1 cup fresh baby spinach**

1. Heat the oil in a small pan over medium-high heat until it is hot enough to make a drop of water dance in the pan. Crack the eggs into the pan and reduce the heat to medium. Fry the eggs until they are done the way you like them.
2. While the eggs are cooking, toast the 2 slices of bread.
3. Spread hummus over both slices of toast. Top 1 slice with a generous handful of spinach and the fried eggs. Place the other slice of toast on top, cut the sandwich in half, and enjoy warm.

NUTRITION PER SERVING

Calories 380 • Fat 19 g • Fiber 7 g • Protein 22 g • Carbohydrates 32 g

# banana shake

MAKES 1 SERVING

1 (6-ounce) container nonfat fruit-flavored yogurt
1 teaspoon honey
1 small banana, peeled and cut into chunks
⅓ cup skim milk
Pinch of cinnamon

Combine all ingredients in a blender and process until smooth.

NUTRITION PER SERVING
Calories 220 • Fat 0 g • Fiber 3 g • Protein 11 g • Carbohydrates 47 g

# peanut butter and banana smoothie

MAKES 1 SERVING

¾ cup very cold skim milk
Ice cubes
⅓ cup milk-chocolate instant breakfast drink mix
½ banana, peeled and cut into chunks
2 tablespoons peanut butter

Measure out the milk in a measuring cup and add enough ice to bring the total to 1 cup; pour into a blender. Add the remaining ingredients and blend until smooth.

NUTRITION PER SERVING
Calories 370 • Fat 19 g • Fiber 4 g • Protein 18 g • Carbohydrates 37 g

## banana hammer smoothie

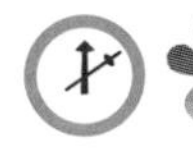

MAKES 2 SERVINGS

- 3 ripe bananas, sliced and frozen
- 2 tablespoons honey
- ½ cup nonfat vanilla or plain yogurt
- ½ cup skim or soy milk (white cranberry or orange juice will work as well)
- 1 cup ice cubes

Combine all ingredients in a blender and process until smooth. If the smoothie is too thick, add more milk to thin.

NUTRITION PER SERVING

Calories 270 • Fat 0.5 g • Fiber 5 g • Protein 7 g • Carbohydrates 65 g

## best banana-blueberry smoothie

MAKES 2 SERVINGS

- 2 bananas, peeled and cut into chunks
- 1 cup frozen blueberries
- 1 (6-ounce) container low-fat blueberry yogurt
- 1 tablespoon packed brown sugar
- 20 whole almonds
- 1 cup skim milk
- 4 ice cubes

Place all ingredients in a blender and process until smooth.

NUTRITION PER SERVING

Calories 350 • Fat 8 g • Fiber 7 g • Protein 12 g • Carbohydrates 61 g

## fruity-o smoothie

MAKES 2 SERVINGS

**1 envelope instant oatmeal (flavored oatmeal, like strawberries and cream, makes a great drink)**
**1 cup skim milk**
**1 large banana, peeled and cut into chunks**
**1 cup frozen strawberries or mixed berries**

Place all ingredients in a blender and process until smooth.

NUTRITION PER SERVING
Calories 210 • Fat 1.5 g • Fiber 5 g • Protein 8 g • Carbohydrates 44 g

## green tea–melon smoothie

MAKES 2 SERVINGS

The astringency of the tea is nicely balanced by the sweetness of the melon and yogurt.

**2 cups cubed honeydew melon**
**1 cup low-fat vanilla yogurt**
**½ teaspoon dried mint**
**½ teaspoon matcha (a type of powdered green tea)**
**Ice cubes**

Place all ingredients in a blender, using enough ice to fill the blender, and process until smooth.

NUTRITION PER SERVING
Calories 190 • Fat 1.5 g • Fiber 2 g • Protein 6 g • Carbohydrates 41 g

# strawberry-blueberry smoothie

MAKES 2 MEAL-SIZE SERVINGS

**1 (32-ounce) container nonfat vanilla yogurt**
**2 cups frozen strawberries**
**1 cup frozen blueberries**
**2 tablespoons flaxseed**

Combine half of all ingredients in a blender and process until smooth. Pour into 1 serving glass; repeat with the remaining ingredients.

NUTRITION PER SERVING
Calories 550 • Fat 1.5 g • Fiber 8 g • Protein 28 g • Carbohydrates 103 g

# banana–wheat germ smoothie

MAKES 1 SERVING

This yummy smoothie is easy to make, full of fiber, and portable — pour it into a travel mug and you can drink it on your way to class. You can substitute other fruit for the banana if you like.

**2 cups skim milk**
**1 ripe banana (overripe banana is fine), peeled and cut into chunks**
**2 tablespoons raw wheat germ**

Combine all ingredients in a blender and blend until smooth.

NUTRITION PER SERVING
Calories 330 • Fat 2.5 g • Fiber 5 g • Protein 21 g • Carbohydrates 58 g

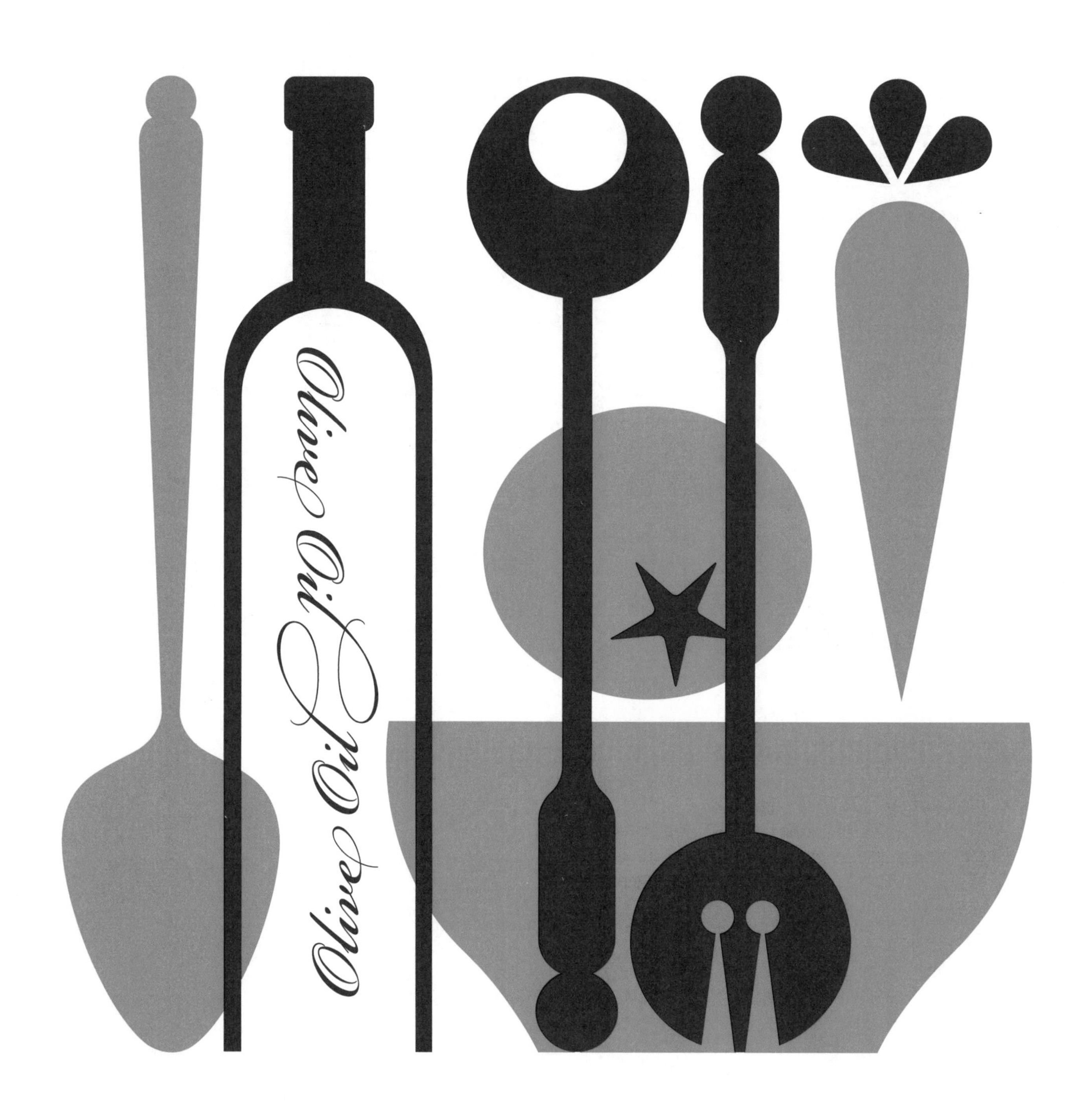
Olive Oil Olive Oil

# chapter 4

## soups & salads

Soups and salads are versatile dishes that can be enjoyed as first courses, healthy snacks, or complete meals. While hot soup is especially welcome on cold winter evenings, we also have some chilled varieties, which provide a refreshing touch on warmer days. Keep in mind that soups often freeze well, so it's a good idea to make extra for quick meals throughout the week.

As for salads, while iceberg lettuce with oil and vinegar is always an option, there are many more interesting combinations that deserve a try. Ingredients can range from greens to pasta to fruit, and even to tofu for the more adventurous. Many of the suggestions offered in this section are as good for large gatherings as they are for solo dinners. Don't worry if you don't have all of the vegetables that a recipe calls for — just use what you have and see how things turn out. You may even like your new salad better.

Try mixing and matching vinaigrettes and dressings with different types of salads. We've included a number of recipes for homemade dressings on pages 115 to 117.

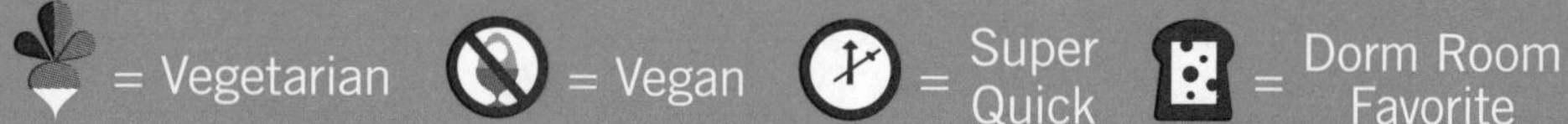
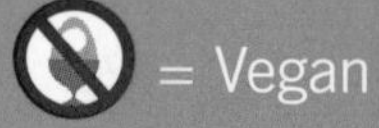
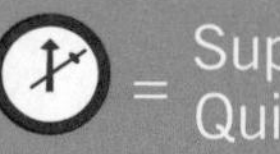
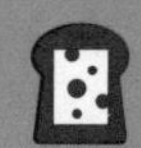

= Vegetarian = Vegan = Super Quick = Dorm Room Favorite

# bean and tomato soup

MAKES 4 SERVINGS, USING 15-OUNCE CANS

This could be the world's easiest soup to make — and it tastes good. It doesn't matter what size cans of tomatoes, beans, and broth you use as long as all three cans are about the same size.

**1 can whole stewed tomatoes, drained and cut into bite-size pieces**
**1 can kidney beans, rinsed and drained**
**1 can low-sodium vegetable broth**
**½ garlic clove, finely chopped**
**A dash of freshly ground black pepper**

1. Combine the contents of the 3 cans in a saucepan. Bring the mixture to a boil, then add the garlic and pepper. Reduce heat and simmer for 10 minutes.
2. Pour half of the mixture into a blender and process until smooth. Return the mixture to the pot, mix well, and serve.

NUTRITION PER SERVING

Calories 130 • Fat 0 g • Fiber 7 g • Protein 7 g • Carbohydrates 26 g

## chilled cucumber dill soup

MAKES 4 SERVINGS

**4 medium cucumbers**
**2 cups nonfat plain yogurt**
**2 tablespoons fresh dill**
**½ teaspoon salt**
**1 teaspoon lemon juice**

1. Slice the cucumbers lengthwise. Scoop out and discard the seeds, then chop the cucumbers.
2. Process all ingredients in a blender until smooth.
3. Refrigerate for 30 minutes. Serve cold.

NUTRITION PER SERVING
Calories 70 • Fat 0 g • Fiber 1 g • Protein 6 g • Carbohydrates 14 g

## egg drop soup

MAKES 6 SERVINGS

**2 (14.5-ounce) cans low-sodium chicken broth**
**2 cups water**
**1 teaspoon ground or freshly grated ginger**
**3 eggs, beaten**
**1 tablespoon sliced scallions**

1. Combine theground broth, water, and ginger in a medium pot. Bring to a boil.
2. Drizzle in the eggs and cook for 1 minute longer. Serve hot, garnish with scallions.

NUTRITION PER SERVING
Calories 60 • Fat 3 g • Fiber 0 g • Protein 6 g • Carbohydrates 3 g

# potato-leek soup

MAKES 6 SERVINGS

If you eat cheese, this soup is very good served with a sprinkle of Parmesan. Be sure to clean your leeks thoroughly — grit often gets caught between the layers. Also, use only the light-colored part of the leek; the green part is tough and not as flavorful.

**3 medium potatoes, peeled and cut into bite-size pieces**
**4 large leeks, chopped (about 3 cups)**
**2 tablespoons finely chopped chives**
**2 medium carrots, peeled and chopped**
**4 cups water**
**1 teaspoon salt**
**Freshly ground black pepper**

1. Place the potatoes, leeks, chives, carrots, water, and salt in a large pot. Bring to a boil, reduce heat, and simmer for 20 minutes, or until the potatoes are tender. Remove from heat and allow the contents to cool until the pot is comfortable to handle.

2. Transfer the soup to a blender or food processor and purée. Return the soup to the pot and heat. Season with pepper to taste and serve.

NUTRITION PER SERVING
Calories 100 • Fat 0 g • Fiber 3 g • Protein 3 g • Carbohydrates 23 g

# zucchini-broccoli soup

MAKES 4 SERVINGS

**1⅓ cups water**
**1½ cups chopped broccoli**
**2 medium zucchini, sliced**
**2 cubes low-sodium chicken bouillon**
**½ teaspoon minced garlic**
**A dash of freshly ground black pepper**

1. Heat the water in a saucepan. Place the broccoli in a steamer insert and steam over the boiling water for 3 minutes. Add the zucchini to the broccoli and steam 1 minute longer. Remove the vegetables from the pan, reserving the steaming water.
2. Drop the bouillon cubes into the water and stir until dissolved.
3. Combine all ingredients (including the bouillon broth) in a blender and purée.

NUTRITION PER SERVING
Calories 50 • Fat 0.5 g • Fiber 3 g • Protein 3 g • Carbohydrates 9 g

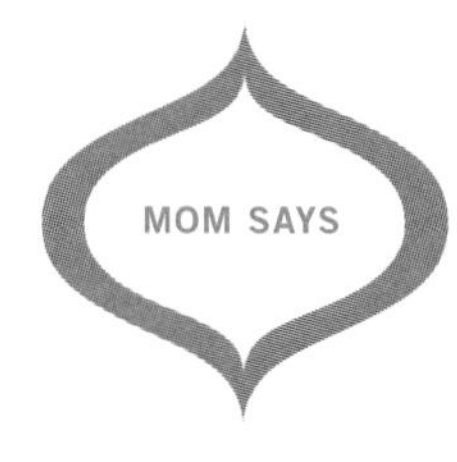


## quick & easy vegetables

To steam any kind of fresh vegetable, first chop it up into whatever size you prefer. Place it in a steamer basket or a stainless-steel colander that will fit inside a pot and fill the pot with an inch or two of water. If you don't have a steamer or colander, you can place the vegetables right in the pot and fill it with just ¼ to ½ inch of water. Bring to a boil, reduce heat, cover the pot, and simmer until the vegetables are tender. Different vegetables take different amounts of time — squash, for example, takes only a minute, while broccoli takes a couple of minutes, and string beans take about five minutes.

# creamy corn and potato chowder

MAKES 2 SERVINGS

When you're baking potatoes for another meal, keep this recipe in mind — it's a very tasty reason to bake extras.

**1 large leftover baked potato, skin removed**
**1 cup low-fat or skim milk**
**1 (15-ounce) can creamed corn**
**2 teaspoons freshly ground black pepper**
**2 teaspoons salt or no-salt seasoning**

1. Mash the potato in a microwave-safe bowl. Stir in the milk, corn, pepper, and salt and mix well.
2. Heat the mixture in a microwave or transfer to a pot and heat on the stovetop. Serve immediately.

NUTRITION PER SERVING
Calories 310 • Fat 1.5 g • Fiber 8 g • Protein 11 g • Carbohydrates 69 g

# black bean–onion soup

MAKES 6 SERVINGS

You can also make this recipe with dried beans; just cook them according to the package directions.

**1 tablespoon canola oil**
**2 small onions, chopped**
**3 garlic cloves, minced**
**2 (15-ounce) cans black beans, rinsed and drained**
**3 cups water**
**1 green bell pepper, seeded and chopped**
**Salt and freshly ground black pepper**

1. Heat the oil in a large pot over medium heat. Add the onions and garlic and sauté until soft, about 7 minutes. Add the beans and water and bring to a boil. Stir in the green pepper. Reduce heat and simmer for 10 minutes.

2. Allow the soup to cool slightly. Transfer half of the soup to a blender and purée. Return the mixture to the pot, season to taste with salt and pepper, and heat to serving temperature.

NUTRITION PER SERVING

Calories 110 • Fat 2.5 g • Fiber 7 g • Protein 6 g • Carbohydrates 22 g

# lentil-corn soup

MAKES 8 SERVINGS

This recipe takes about an hour to prepare, but most of the work is nothing more than keeping an eye on the pot. The soup is great served with a hearty bread.

**1 cup dried lentils, rinsed**
**4 cups water**
**1 medium onion, chopped**
**2 cups chopped tomatoes, fresh or canned**
**2 cups corn kernels, fresh or frozen**
**1 teaspoon dried basil**
**3 garlic cloves, minced**
**1½ teaspoons salt**

1. Combine the lentils and water in a large pot. Bring to a boil, reduce heat, and simmer for 30 to 40 minutes, or until the lentils are soft.
2. Add the remaining ingredients, and simmer for 20 minutes longer. Serve hot.

NUTRITION PER SERVING

Calories 150 • Fat 0.5 g • Fiber 5 g • Protein 9 g • Carbohydrates 27 g

# butternut-quinoa soup

MAKES 4 SERVINGS

This is an inexpensive, deliciously creamy soup. With bread and salad, it makes a great fall or winter dinner.

- **1 medium butternut squash**
- **4 cups water**
- **½ teaspoon salt**
- **1 apple, peeled, cored, and chopped**
- **2 medium carrots, peeled and chopped**
- **½ cup chopped onion**
- **1 cup quinoa or rice**
- **1 cup plain yogurt**
- **½ teaspoon freshly ground black pepper**
- **½ teaspoon curry powder**
- **½ teaspoon dried thyme**

1. Cut the squash in half and remove the seeds. Peel the squash; you can use a peeler, but sometimes it's easier to pare off the skin with a sharp knife. Chop the orange-yellow flesh into 1-inch chunks. Place in a large pot and cover with the water. Bring to a boil, add salt, reduce heat, and simmer, covered, for 20 minutes.

2. Add the apple, carrots, and onion. Continue to simmer over medium heat until all are soft, about 10 minutes. Drain, reserving 2 cups of the cooking liquid.

3. In a separate pot, cook the quinoa according to the package directions. (If you buy the quinoa in bulk, without directions for cooking it, just cook it like rice: Bring twice as much water to a boil, add the grains, and simmer until the liquid is absorbed and the grains are tender.)

4. Use a food processor, blender, or immersion blender to purée the squash mixture. Pour the purée back into your large pot, add the reserved cooking liquid, yogurt, pepper, curry powder, and thyme, and cook over low heat, stirring constantly, until all the ingredients are hot and thoroughly combined. Stir in the quinoa and serve.

NUTRITION PER SERVING

Calories 240 • Fat 3 g • Fiber 6 g • Protein 10 g • Carbohydrates 46 g

# thai coconut–red curry soup

MAKES 6 SERVINGS

This delicious, spicy soup is quite flexible — you can add whatever vegetables or meat you prefer. It tastes even better when warmed up again the next day!

- **2 (13.5-ounce) cans light coconut milk**
- **1 (32-ounce) container low-sodium chicken broth**
- **2 tablespoons packed brown sugar**
- **1 teaspoon to 1 tablespoon red curry paste (depending on how spicy you like it)**
- **1 tablespoon fish sauce**
- **1 teaspoon sesame oil**
- **1 pound shredded cooked chicken or cubed tofu (optional)**
- **1 sweet potato, diced (optional)**
- **1 small zucchini, chopped (optional)**
- **1 (8-ounce) can bamboo shoots, drained (optional)**
- **1 (8-ounce) can sliced water chestnuts, drained (optional)**
- **1 tablespoon lime juice**
- **2 portobello mushrooms, sliced**
- **3 scallions, chopped**
- **1 pound cooked shrimp**

1. Shake up the cans of coconut milk (sometimes the fat separates from the rest of the liquid) before opening them. Combine the coconut milk, broth, sugar, curry paste, fish sauce, and sesame oil in a large pot. Bring to a simmer over medium-low heat. Add the chicken, sweet potato, zucchini, bamboo shoots, and/or water chestnuts, if you're using them, and simmer for 15 to 20 minutes.
2. About 5 minutes before serving, stir the lime juice, mushrooms, and scallions into the soup. Add the shrimp just before serving. Serve hot.

NUTRITION PER SERVING

Calories 390 • Fat 15 g • Fiber 2 g • Protein 22 g • Carbohydrates 13 g

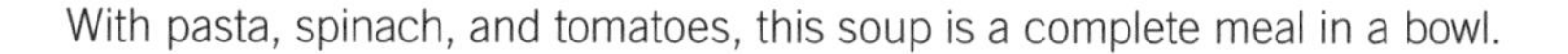

# tortellini soup

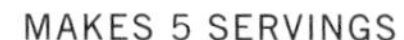

MAKES 5 SERVINGS

With pasta, spinach, and tomatoes, this soup is a complete meal in a bowl.

**1 tablespoon extra-virgin olive oil**
**2 garlic cloves, minced**
**3 (14.5-ounce) cans low-sodium vegetable or chicken broth**
**1 (9-ounce) package refrigerated cheese tortellini**
**1 (10-ounce) package frozen chopped spinach, thawed and squeezed dry**
**1 (14.5-ounce) can diced tomatoes with green chiles, undrained**
**Sliced mushrooms (optional)**

1. Heat the oil in a pot over medium heat. Add the garlic and sauté 2 minutes, until just golden.
2. Stir in the broth and bring to a boil. Add the tortellini and cook for 5 to 6 minutes, until tender. Stir in the spinach, tomatoes, and mushrooms, if using, and heat until warmed through. Serve hot.

NUTRITION PER SERVING

Calories 240 • Fat 7 g • Fiber 4 g • Protein 9 g • Carbohydrates 32 g

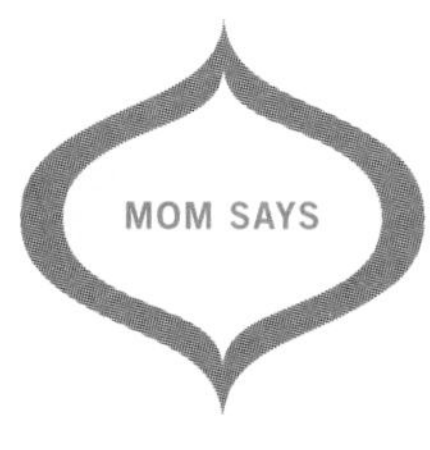


## cooking with broth

- When an otherwise all-vegetable recipe calls for beef or chicken broth, you can substitute vegetable broth to make the recipe vegetarian.
- Many canned broths and bouillon cubes are extremely high in sodium, so when you're shopping, be sure to look for the low-sodium varieties.

# mama bahr's carrot soup

MAKES 4 SERVINGS

This soup is terrific, hot or cold.

- 2 tablespoons butter
- ½ large onion, minced
- 2 (14.5-ounce) cans low-sodium vegetable or chicken broth
- 1½ tablespoons tomato paste
- ¼ cup rice
- ¾ pound carrots, peeled and chopped
- Salt and freshly ground black pepper

1. Melt the butter in a large pot over medium heat. Sauté the onion in the butter until it is translucent.
2. Add the broth, tomato paste, rice, and carrots to the sautéed onion. Bring to a boil, reduce heat, and simmer until the carrots are soft, about 45 minutes.
3. Purée the soup in a blender or food processor. (You may need to do it in a couple of batches.) Season with salt and pepper to taste. Serve hot or cold.

NUTRITION PER SERVING

Calories 140 • Fat 6 g • Fiber 3 g • Protein 2 g • Carbohydrates 18 g

# gazpacho

MAKES 6 SERVINGS

Although this recipe has many ingredients, it takes only about 20 minutes to make. Gazpacho is best in the summer when tomatoes are fresh and full of flavor. If you prefer smooth gazpacho, rather than chunky, simply purée the finished recipe.

**1 (14.5-ounce) can low-sodium vegetable broth**
**2 cups tomato juice**
**2 tablespoons lemon juice**
**½ teaspoon hot sauce**
**1 garlic clove, minced**
**1 teaspoon salt**
**1 green bell pepper, seeded and chopped**
**1 cucumber, peeled, seeded, and chopped**
**4 medium tomatoes, chopped**
**1 onion, chopped**

1. Combine the broth, tomato juice, lemon juice, hot sauce, garlic, and salt in a large pot over medium heat. Heat, uncovered, until the mixture comes to a boil.
2. Add the green pepper, cucumber, tomatoes, and onion. Return to a boil, reduce heat, and simmer for 2 minutes. Remove from heat.
3. Cover and refrigerate. Serve cold.

NUTRITION PER SERVING
Calories 60 • Fat 0 g • Fiber 3 g • Protein 2 g • Carbohydrates 13 g

# mushroom-barley soup

MAKES 6 SERVINGS

Barley is a tasty and healthy grain. You can find it in the grains section of any grocery store.

**1 tablespoon butter**
**½ large yellow onion, finely chopped**
**1 small carrot, peeled and finely chopped**
**1 small celery stalk, finely chopped**
**15 medium white mushrooms, wiped clean and chopped**
**3 (14.5-ounce) cans low-sodium vegetable, chicken, or beef broth**
**1 cup pearl barley, rinsed**
**Salt and freshly ground black pepper**

1. Melt the butter in a large pot over medium heat. Add the onion, carrot, and celery and sauté until the onion is translucent. Add the mushrooms and cook until they begin to soften.
2. Add the broth and barley to the sautéed vegetables. Bring to a boil, reduce heat, and simmer for 50 to 60 minutes, or until the barley is tender. Season with salt and pepper to taste.

NUTRITION PER SERVING

Calories 80 • Fat 2 g • Fiber 2 g • Protein 1 g • Carbohydrates 13 g

# quick veggie soup

MAKES 6 SERVINGS

This soup could not be any easier to make, but the best part about it is its versatility. Although it works best if you can include some carrot or potato, use whatever vegetables you have on hand. Make it vegan by substituting olive oil for the butter.

**½ tablespoon butter**
**1 yellow onion, chopped**
**2 medium carrots, peeled and chopped**
**2 (14.5-ounce) cans low-sodium vegetable or chicken broth**
**1 celery stalk, chopped**
**1 cup chopped broccoli**
**½ baking potato, peeled and chopped**
**½ teaspoon dried oregano**
**Salt and freshly ground black pepper**

1. Melt the butter in a large pot over medium heat. Add the onion and carrots and sauté until the onion is translucent.
2. Add the broth, celery, broccoli, potato, oregano, and salt and pepper to taste. Bring to a boil, reduce heat, and simmer for 20 minutes or until the potato is tender.

NUTRITION PER SERVING
Calories 70 • Fat 1 g • Fiber 3 g • Protein 2 g • Carbohydrates 13 g

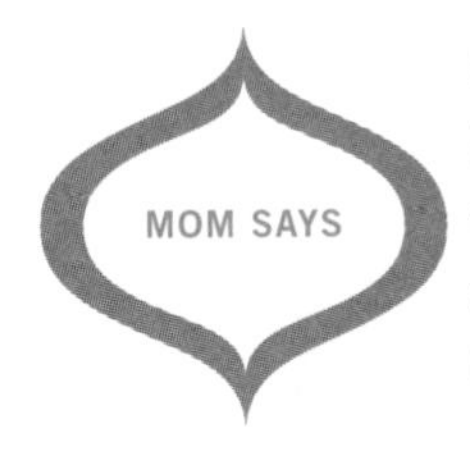


## saving soup

Freezing soup is a great way to plan for the upcoming week. However, don't fill the container to the brim. As soup freezes it will expand, so you'll need to leave some headroom.

# onion soup

MAKES 6 SERVINGS

This is an elegant and incredibly cheap soup. The plain soup can be a light lunch or first course for dinner. Make it a meal by floating a slice of toasted French bread topped with melted Gruyère cheese in the bowl and serving a green salad on the side.

**2 tablespoons butter**
**3 medium onions, thinly sliced**
**6 cups low-sodium chicken broth**
**¼ teaspoon freshly ground black pepper**

1. Melt the butter in a large pot over medium heat. Add the onions and sauté until they are deep brown, 12 to 15 minutes.
2. Add the broth and pepper. Bring the mixture to a boil, reduce heat, and simmer for 20 minutes. Serve hot.

NUTRITION PER SERVING
Calories 90 • Fat 5 g • Fiber 1 g • Protein 5 g • Carbohydrates 8 g

# quick chicken soup

MAKES 3 SERVINGS

This soup is a great way to use up leftover chicken. If you prefer an even heartier soup, try adding some rice or pasta. If the rice or pasta is uncooked, add it to the boiling water with the other ingredients in step one; if it's already cooked, add it five minutes before the soup is done cooking.

**3 cups water**
**3 cubes low-sodium chicken bouillon**
**2 carrots, peeled and sliced**
**2 celery stalks, chopped**
**1 cup chopped cooked chicken**

1. Bring the water to a boil in a medium saucepan. Add the bouillon cubes, carrots, and celery, return to a boil, then reduce heat and simmer for 10 minutes, or until the carrots are soft.
2. Add the chicken and simmer for 2 minutes longer.

NUTRITION PER SERVING
Calories 160 • Fat 6 g • Fiber 1 g • Protein 18 g • Carbohydrates 8 g

## basic green salad

  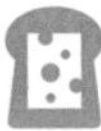

MAKES 4 SERVINGS

**½ head lettuce (try using more than one variety), or 1 (16-ounce) bag salad greens**
**1 plump tomato, sliced**
**⅓ red onion, thinly sliced**

Wash, dry, and chop the lettuce. Place in a serving bowl and top with the tomato and onion. Serve with your favorite dressing.

NUTRITION PER SERVING

Calories 20 • Fat 0 g • Fiber 1 g • Protein 1 g • Carbohydrates 4 g

## mediterranean salad

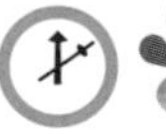  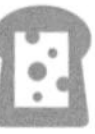

MAKES 4 SERVINGS

**1 large tomato, chopped**
**½ cucumber, halved lengthwise and sliced**
**¾ cup shredded low-fat mozzarella cheese**
**¼ cup olives, pitted and halved**
**¾ (15-ounce) can chickpeas, rinsed and drained**
**⅓ cup Italian dressing (see page 115 for our recipe)**
**Dried oregano**

Combine the tomato, cucumber, cheese, olives, and chickpeas. Add the dressing and toss lightly. Sprinkle with oregano to taste.

NUTRITION PER SERVING

Calories 420 • Fat 15 g • Fiber 15 g • Protein 22 g • Carbohydrates 53 g

# greek salad

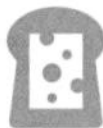

MAKES 4 SERVINGS

Oregano, lemon, and feta give this salad its bright Greek flavor. It's substantial enough to be dinner.

- **2 heads romaine lettuce**
- **½ red onion, chopped**
- **1 cucumber, chopped**
- **1 green bell pepper, seeded and chopped**
- **1 tomato, cut into wedges**
- **¼ cup crumbled feta cheese**
- **⅓ cup pitted and sliced black olives**
- **2 tablespoons extra-virgin olive oil**
- **2 tablespoons lemon juice**
- **1 tablespoon red wine vinegar**
- **1 garlic clove, minced**
- **1 teaspoon chopped fresh oregano or ½ teaspoon dried**
- **Salt and freshly ground black pepper**

1. Toss the lettuce, onion, cucumber, green pepper, tomato, feta, and olives in a large bowl.
2. In a separate bowl, whisk together the olive oil, lemon juice, vinegar, garlic, oregano, and salt and pepper to taste.
3. Pour the dressing over the salad and toss. Serve immediately.

NUTRITION PER SERVING

Calories 140 • Fat 10 g • Fiber 3 g • Protein 3 g • Carbohydrates 10 g

# bok choy salad

MAKES 4 SERVINGS

Because bok choy is a mild member of the cabbage family, this salad is a nice cross between a green salad and cole slaw.

**1 large head bok choy**
**1 large onion, chopped**
**½ cup shelled sunflower seeds**
**½ cup slivered almonds**
**3 packages ramen noodles, crumbled (throw the seasoning packets away)**
**4 tablespoons butter, melted**
**3 tablespoons low-sodium soy sauce**
**¼ cup rice vinegar**
**½ cup canola oil**
**½ cup sugar**

1. Preheat the oven to 450°F.
2. Separate the bok choy leaves, cutting off the thickest part of the stem. Wash thoroughly and dry. Chop the stems and leaves into bite-size pieces. Toss the bok choy and onions in a large bowl.
3. Place the sunflower seeds, almonds, and noodles in a separate bowl. Pour butter over the mixture; blend well. Transfer the mixture to a baking sheet and bake for 3 to 5 minutes. Watch closely; stir after 2 minutes.
4. Pour the soy sauce, vinegar, oil, and sugar into a jar with a tight-fitting lid. Shake thoroughly to blend.
5. Toss the dressing to taste with the bok choy and onions. Let sit for at least 10 minutes before serving. When you are ready to eat, sprinkle the seed mixture over the salad and serve.

NUTRITION PER SERVING
Calories 840 • Fat 53 g • Fiber 10 g • Protein 16 g • Carbohydrates 82 g

# chicken caesar salad with cranberries

MAKES 1 SERVING

The cranberries and tart apple add a great punch to the creamy flavor of the Caesar dressing.

- **1½ cups coarsely chopped romaine lettuce**
- **1 cup loosely packed spinach leaves**
- **½ cup grape tomatoes**
- **¼ cup grated Parmesan cheese**
- **¼ cup sliced red onion**
- **¼ cup peeled and diced Granny Smith apple**
- **¼ cup dried cranberries**
- **¼ cup low-fat Caesar salad dressing**
- **1 boneless, skinless chicken breast half, cooked and sliced**

Combine romaine, spinach, tomatoes, Parmesan, onion, apple, and cranberries in a serving bowl. Add Caesar dressing and toss to coat. Top with sliced chicken.

NUTRITION PER SERVING

Calories 710 • Fat 26 g • Fiber 9 g • Protein 20 g • Carbohydrates 50 g

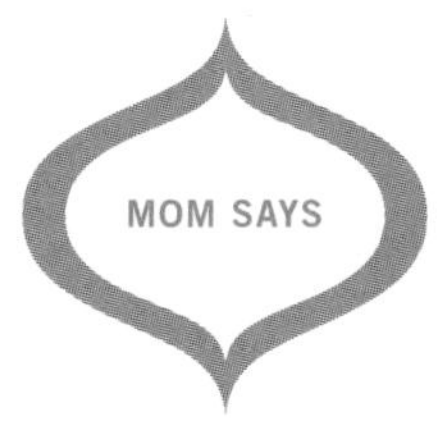


## making croutons

Make your own croutons for salads by cutting French bread into small cubes. Dry the cubes on a cookie sheet in a 200°F oven until brown and crunchy. It's a great way to use up bread that's going stale.

# roasted red pepper and feta salad

MAKES 4 SERVINGS

Substitute tomatoes for the roasted red peppers for an equally tasty salad.

**1 roasted red pepper, chopped (see page 53)**
**½ cup crumbled feta cheese**
**½ teaspoon dried oregano**
**½ head lettuce, washed and chopped**

Combine the pepper and the cheese, tossing to mix. Season with oregano. Serve on a bed of lettuce.

NUTRITION PER SERVING
Calories 60 • Fat 4 g • Fiber 1 g • Protein 3 g • Carbohydrates 3 g

# tomato, basil, and mozzarella

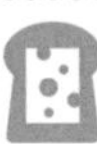

MAKES 4 SERVINGS

Fresh mozzarella is packed in liquid and usually comes in a ball; it's not the same as the grated mozzarella that you put on pizza.

**4 slices tomato**
**4 leaves fresh basil**
**4 slices fresh mozzarella**
**4 teaspoons extra-virgin olive oil**
**Sea salt and freshly ground black pepper**

Place the tomatoes on a plate. Top each slice with a basil leaf and slice of mozzarella. Sprinkle with oil and salt and pepper to taste.

NUTRITION PER SERVING
Calories 90 • Fat 6 g • Fiber 0 g • Protein 7 g • Carbohydrates 2 g

# salad caprese

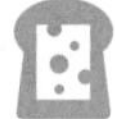

MAKES 4 SERVINGS

In contrast to plain tomato, basil, and mozzarella, this traditional Italian salad has a vinegar kick.

**1 ball of fresh mozzarella (about ½ pound)**
**2 ripe tomatoes (Roma tomatoes work especially well)**
**Fresh basil leaves**
**Sea salt**
**Freshly ground black pepper**
**Balsamic vinegar**
**Extra-virgin olive oil**

1. Cut the mozzarella and tomatoes into ¼-inch-thick slices.
2. Place a mozzarella slice on a platter, and top with a tomato slice and a basil leaf. Repeat with remaining cheese, tomato, and basil. Sprinkle lightly with salt and pepper. Drizzle each stack with a little bit of balsamic vinegar and olive oil.

NUTRITION PER SERVING
Calories 210 • Fat 13 g • Fiber 1 g • Protein 16 g • Carbohydrates 6 g

# red lentil-beet salad

MAKES 4 SERVINGS

This is a delicious salad — colorful and packed with nutrition. You might want to roast extra beets and add them to other salads or just eat them out of the fridge.

**4 beets**
**¼ cup olive oil**
**2 tablespoons balsamic vinegar**
**1 tablespoon fresh lemon juice**
**½ teaspoon cumin**
**Salt and freshly ground pepper**
**1 cup red lentils**
**1 large bunch arugula, trimmed and washed**
**2½ ounces goat cheese, crumbled**

1. Preheat the oven to 350°F.
2. Wrap the beets in foil and roast them until they are tender, about 45 minutes. When the beets are cool enough to handle, peel them and cut into ½-inch pieces.
3. Combine the oil, vinegar, lemon juice, cumin, and salt and pepper to taste; stir well.
4. Bring a medium pot of water to a boil. Add the lentils and cook for about 10 minutes, just until the lentils are tender. Drain, and mix in half of the vinaigrette. Let cool.
5. Toss the arugula and beets with the remaining vinaigrette.
6. Divide the arugula and beets among 4 plates. Top with a few spoonfuls of lentils and some goat cheese.

NUTRITION PER SERVING

Calories 390 • Fat 19 g • Fiber 10 g • Protein 18 g • Carbohydrates 39 g

# taco salad

MAKES 4 SERVINGS

This is a hearty salad that should be eaten as a meal.

- **½ pound lean ground beef**
- **Cayenne pepper**
- **Chili powder**
- **Salt and freshly ground black pepper**
- **24 baked corn chips**
- **¼ head lettuce, shredded**
- **1 tomato, chopped**
- **¼ green bell pepper, seeded and finely chopped**
- **3 tablespoons finely chopped red onion**
- **⅓ cup salsa**
- **4 olives, pitted and thinly sliced**

1. Brown the beef in a small skillet over medium heat, stirring to break up the meat. Season with cayenne, chili powder, and salt and pepper to taste. Drain any grease.
2. Divide the chips among 4 shallow bowls. Add one-quarter of the lettuce to the bowls and top each serving with one-quarter of the meat, tomato, green pepper, onion, salsa, and sliced olives.

NUTRITION PER SERVING

Calories 130 • Fat 3.5 g • Fiber 2 g • Protein 13 g • Carbohydrates 12 g

# chicken chow mein salad

MAKES 4 SERVINGS

If you're not planning to serve four portions of this dish at once, dress only the amount you intend to serve. Store the rest of the salad and dressing in the refrigerator until you're ready to have more.

**3 heads romaine lettuce, roughly chopped**
**5 cups broccoli florets**
**1 cup chow mein noodles**
**4 scallions, chopped**
**½ cup vegetable oil**
**¼ cup white wine vinegar**
**¼ cup sugar**
**½ teaspoon soy sauce**
**¼ teaspoon minced garlic**
**Salt and freshly ground black pepper**
**4 boneless, skinless chicken breasts halves, grilled and diced**
**1 cup slivered almonds**

1. Combine the lettuce, broccoli, chow mein noodles, and scallions in a large bowl and set aside.
2. To prepare the dressing, whisk the oil into the vinegar. Add the sugar, soy sauce, and garlic and whisk until blended. Season to taste with salt and pepper.
3. Dress the salad greens with the dressing. Top with the chicken and almonds.

NUTRITION PER SERVING

Calories 650 • Fat 47 g • Fiber 8 g • Protein 24 g • Carbohydrates 40 g

# bok choy salad with nut-crusted chicken

MAKES 2 SERVINGS

Insanely delicious and incredibly easy!

**2 heads baby bok choy, chopped**
**3 scallions, finely chopped**
**1 handful mixed nuts, such as almonds and peanuts, whole**
**Salt and freshly ground black pepper**
**1 egg**
**¼ cup all-purpose flour**
**1 handful mixed nuts, finely chopped**
**2 tablespoons extra-virgin olive oil**
**2 boneless, skinless chicken breast halves, pounded thin**
**¼ cup chopped onion**
**¼ red bell pepper, seeded and chopped**
**1 garlic clove, minced**
**2 tablespoons prepared Asian-style sesame salad dressing**

1. Toss the bok choy, scallions, and whole nuts in a large salad bowl. Lightly season with salt and pepper. Set aside.
2. Beat the egg with a splash of water in a shallow bowl. Combine the flour with liberal amounts of salt and pepper in a separate shallow bowl. Mix in the chopped nuts.
3. Heat 1 tablespoon of the olive oil in a large skillet over medium heat. Dip the chicken in the egg wash, dredge them in the flour mixture, and drop them into the skillet. Sauté the fillets for about 2 minutes on each side, or until the outsides are golden brown.
4. While the chicken is cooking, heat the remaining 1 tablespoon olive oil in a medium skillet over medium heat. Add the onion, red pepper, and garlic and sauté for about 2 minutes, until they just begin to soften. Season with salt and pepper to taste.
5. Slice the chicken fillets into thin strips. Top the bok choy mixture with the chicken and sautéed vegetables. Drizzle with the sesame dressing and enjoy.

NUTRITION PER SERVING

Calories 720 • Fat 45 g • Fiber 14 g • Protein 46 g • Carbohydrates 45 g

# potato salad

MAKES 4 SERVINGS

The skin of a potato contains quite a bit of its nutritional value, so don't peel your potatoes before cooking them unless the skin is particularly thick — you'll be throwing away the best part of the dish.

**4 medium red potatoes, washed**
**¼ cup red wine vinegar**
**2 tablespoons water**
**1 teaspoon lemon juice**
**1 teaspoon extra-virgin olive oil**
**2 tablespoons fresh dill**
**3 tablespoons chopped onion**
**1 teaspoon sugar**
**½ teaspoon salt**
**Pinch of freshly ground black pepper**

1. Place the potatoes in a large pot with enough cold water just to cover. Bring to a boil, salt the water, and cook for 20 to 30 minutes, or until tender when pierced with a knife.
2. Remove the potatoes from the water and let cool. Slice the potatoes into ½-inch-thick slices and place in a large bowl.
3. Mix together the vinegar, water, lemon juice, oil, dill, onion, sugar, salt, and pepper. Pour over the potatoes and let sit for several minutes before serving.

NUTRITION PER SERVING
Calories 170 • Fat 1.5 g • Fiber 3 g • Protein 4 g • Carbohydrates 36 g

# fruit salad

MAKES 4 SERVINGS

A great summer and spring salad.

- **2 medium apples, cored, peeled, and chopped**
- **1 tangerine, peeled and sectioned**
- **1 cup halved seedless green grapes**
- **½ cup sliced strawberries**
- **1 tablespoon chopped fresh mint**
- **1 cup nonfat plain yogurt**

Combine all ingredients in a large bowl and mix well. For best flavor, cover and refrigerate overnight.

NUTRITION PER SERVING

Calories 130 • Fat 0 g • Fiber 4 g • Protein 4 g • Carbohydrates 31 g

# mandarin orange and mint salad

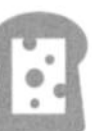

MAKES 4 SERVINGS

This makes a light and delicious salad that's great for the spring or summer months. When you serve it, make sure plenty of mint and orange go into each bowl.

- **1 head romaine lettuce, washed and chopped**
- **1 tablespoon finely chopped fresh mint**
- **3 mandarin oranges, peeled and sectioned**

Combine all ingredients and toss well.

NUTRITION PER SERVING

Calories 45 • Fat 0 g • Fiber 3 g • Protein 2 g • Carbohydrates 13 g

# quick pasta salad

MAKES 10 SERVINGS

This recipe will make enough to serve a crowd. If you're cooking just for yourself, halve the ingredients and save the leftovers for quick lunches and snacks.

**1 (16-ounce) box tricolor pasta (we recommend fusilli)**
**1 cup chopped broccoli**
**2 carrots, peeled and chopped**
**1 onion, thinly sliced**
**1 red bell pepper, seeded and chopped**
**1 cucumber, peeled and sliced**
**¾ cup Italian dressing (see page 115 for our recipe)**

1. Bring a large pot of water to a boil. Salt the water and add the pasta; cook until tender, about 8 minutes. Drain and rinse with cold water.
2. While the pasta is cooking, combine the broccoli, carrots, onion, and red pepper in a microwave-safe dish. Microwave on high for 3 minutes. (If you don't have a microwave, blanch the vegetables.)
3. Combine the cooked vegetables and cucumber with the pasta. Cover and refrigerate until chilled.
4. Pour dressing over the salad when you're ready to serve. Toss to coat.

NUTRITION PER SERVING

Calories 240 • Fat 6 g • Fiber 3 g • Protein 7 g • Carbohydrates 41 g

## bean and corn salad

 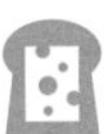

MAKES 4 SERVINGS

**2 (15-ounce) cans black beans, rinsed and drained**
**1 cup frozen corn kernels, rinsed and thawed**
**½ cup thinly sliced red onion**
**1 tomato, diced**
**2 tablespoons cider vinegar**

Combine all ingredients in a large bowl and mix well. Cover and refrigerate. Serve chilled.

NUTRITION PER SERVING
Calories 170 • Fat 0 g • Fiber 12 g • Protein 10 g • Carbohydrates 41 g

## green bean salad

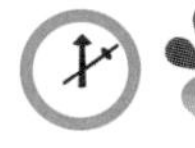 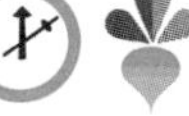

MAKES 4 SERVINGS

A scrumptious way to get your vegetables, this salad works equally well with French, ranch, or vinaigrette dressing, but our own Dijon Salad Dressing is perfect.

**1 pound fresh green beans**
**⅓ cup thinly sliced red onion**
**¼ cup salad dressing of choice (we recommend our Dijon Salad Dressing on page 116)**

1. Wash the green beans and snip off their ends.
2. Bring a large pot of water to a boil. Drop in the green beans and boil for 4 minutes. Drain and rinse in cold water.
3. Toss the onion with the beans and add salad dressing to taste.

NUTRITION PER SERVING
Calories 130 • Fat 4.5 g • Fiber 9 g • Protein 8 g • Carbohydrates 23 g

## coleslaw

MAKES 4 SERVINGS

**¼ head green cabbage, shredded**
**1 carrot, peeled and shredded**
**¼ cup finely chopped red onion**
**¼ cup vinaigrette**
**2 tablespoons nonfat plain yogurt**
**1 tablespoon cider vinegar**
**Salt and freshly ground black pepper to taste**

Mix all ingredients well. Refrigerate until ready to serve.

NUTRITION PER SERVING
Calories 80 • Fat 4 g • Fiber 3 g • Protein 2 g • Carbohydrates 10 g

## egg salad

MAKES 1 SERVING

Serve on lettuce as a salad or in a pita pocket as a sandwich.

**1 hard-boiled egg**
**1 tablespoon nonfat plain yogurt**
**½ teaspoon Dijon mustard**
**Salt and freshly ground black pepper**

Finely chop the egg. Thoroughly mix the chopped egg with the yogurt and mustard. Season to taste with salt and pepper.

NUTRITION PER SERVING
Calories 90 • Fat 5 g • Fiber 0 g • Protein 7 g • Carbohydrates 2 g

## chicken salad

MAKES 4 SERVINGS

Serve over salad greens or as a sandwich filling.

**2 cups chopped cooked chicken**
**¼ cup nonfat plain yogurt**
**2 teaspoons mustard**
**3 tablespoons chopped celery**
**¼ cup chopped seedless green grapes**
**Salt and freshly ground black pepper**

Combine all ingredients and stir until well mixed. Refrigerate or serve immediately.

**NUTRITION PER SERVING**
Calories 200 • Fat 8 g • Fiber 0 g • Protein 27 g • Carbohydrates 4 g

## tuna salad

 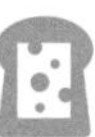

MAKES 2 SERVINGS

Serve on greens or in a sandwich — this salad is tasty either way. Makes great leftovers.

**1 (6-ounce) can water-packed tuna, drained**
**2 tablespoons nonfat plain yogurt**
**½ teaspoon Dijon mustard**
**¼ medium carrot, grated**
**Salt and freshly ground black pepper**

Combine all ingredients and mix well. Refrigerate or serve immediately.

**NUTRITION PER SERVING**
Calories 120 • Fat 2.5 g • Fiber 0 g • Protein 21 g • Carbohydrates 2 g

# chicken-bulgur salad with cranberry vinaigrette

MAKES 4 SERVINGS

To make this salad vegetarian, substitute vegetable broth for the chicken broth and drained black beans for the chicken.

- **1½ cups low-sodium chicken broth**
- **1 cup dry bulgur**
- **2 cups chopped cooked chicken (rotisserie chicken is fine)**
- **1 cup chickpeas, rinsed and drained**
- **1 cup cherry or grape tomatoes (halve them if they're large)**
- **1 cup peeled, finely chopped cucumber**
- **3 scallions, finely chopped (white and light green parts only)**
- **1 cup small black pitted olives**
- **3 tablespoons dried cranberries**
- **3 tablespoons finely chopped fresh parsley**
- **3 tablespoons lime juice**
- **2 tablespoons cranberry juice concentrate (you can buy this frozen and let it thaw)**
- **¼ cup extra-virgin olive oil**

1. Bring the broth to a boil. Pour the hot broth over the bulgur in a large heatproof bowl and stir to blend. Cover and set aside for 30 to 40 minutes, or until the grains have absorbed all of the broth.
2. Stir the bulgur with a fork to fluff it up. Add the chicken, chickpeas, tomatoes, cucumber, scallions, olives, cranberries, and parsley. Toss to blend. Set aside.
3. Combine the lime juice and cranberry juice in a small bowl. Gradually whisk in the olive oil to emulsify. Pour over the chicken mixture and toss to blend. Serve the salad chilled or at room temperature.

NUTRITION PER SERVING

Calories 720 • Fat 30 g • Fiber 17 g • Protein 43 g • Carbohydrates 74 g

## basic oil and vinegar dressing

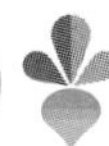

MAKES 6 SERVINGS

- ¼ cup balsamic vinegar
- ¼ cup extra-virgin olive oil
- ¼ cup water
- 1 garlic clove, minced
- ½ teaspoon dried basil
- ½ teaspoon dried oregano
- Salt and freshly ground black pepper

Whisk together all ingredients.

NUTRITION PER SERVING

Calories 100 • Fat 9 g • Fiber 0 g • Protein 0 g • Carbohydrates 3 g

## italian dressing

MAKES 6 SERVINGS

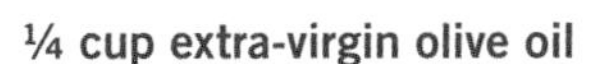

- ¼ cup extra-virgin olive oil
- 3 tablespoons water
- 2 tablespoons white wine vinegar
- 1 garlic clove, minced
- 1 teaspoon dried oregano
- ½ teaspoon Dijon mustard
- Salt and freshly ground black pepper

Whisk together all ingredients.

NUTRITION PER SERVING

Calories 100 • Fat 9 g • Fiber 0 g • Protein 0 g • Carbohydrates 3 g

# dijon salad dressing

MAKES 6 SERVINGS

**2 tablespoons red wine vinegar**
**2 tablespoons balsamic vinegar**
**2 tablespoons Dijon mustard**
**2 tablespoons extra-virgin olive oil**
**Salt and freshly ground black pepper**

Whisk together all ingredients.

NUTRITION PER SERVING
Calories 100 • Fat 4.5 g • Fiber 0 g • Protein 0 g • Carbohydrates 3 g

# blue cheese dressing

MAKES 6 SERVINGS

**¼ cup crumbled blue cheese**
**½ cup nonfat plain yogurt**
**½ garlic clove, minced**
**½ teaspoon Dijon mustard**

Mash half of the cheese in a small bowl. Mix in the yogurt, garlic, and mustard. Add the remaining cheese and stir well.

NUTRITION PER SERVING
Calories 30 • Fat 1.5 g • Fiber 0 g • Protein 2 g • Carbohydrates 2 g

## honey-mustard dressing

MAKES 3 SERVINGS

**2 tablespoons honey**
**1 tablespoon cider vinegar**
**1 tablespoon Dijon mustard**
**1 tablespoon extra-virgin olive oil**
**1 tablespoon water**
**½ teaspoon lemon juice**

Combine all ingredients and mix well. (If the honey is too thick to mix easily, heat it in the microwave for 5 to 10 seconds.)

NUTRITION PER SERVING
Calories 90 • Fat 4.5 g • Fiber 0 g • Protein 0 g • Carbohydrates 12 g

## orange vinaigrette

MAKES 5 SERVINGS

**1 garlic clove, minced**
**1½ tablespoons chopped fresh parsley**
**2 tablespoons white vinegar**
**1 teaspoon sugar**
**½ teaspoon salt**
**⅓ cup orange juice**
**2 tablespoons extra-virgin olive oil**

Combine the garlic and parsley in a small bowl. Add the vinegar, sugar, and salt; mix well. Gradually add the orange juice and oil, whisking constantly.

NUTRITION PER SERVING
Calories 65 • Fat 5 g • Fiber 0 g • Protein 0 g • Carbohydrates 4 g

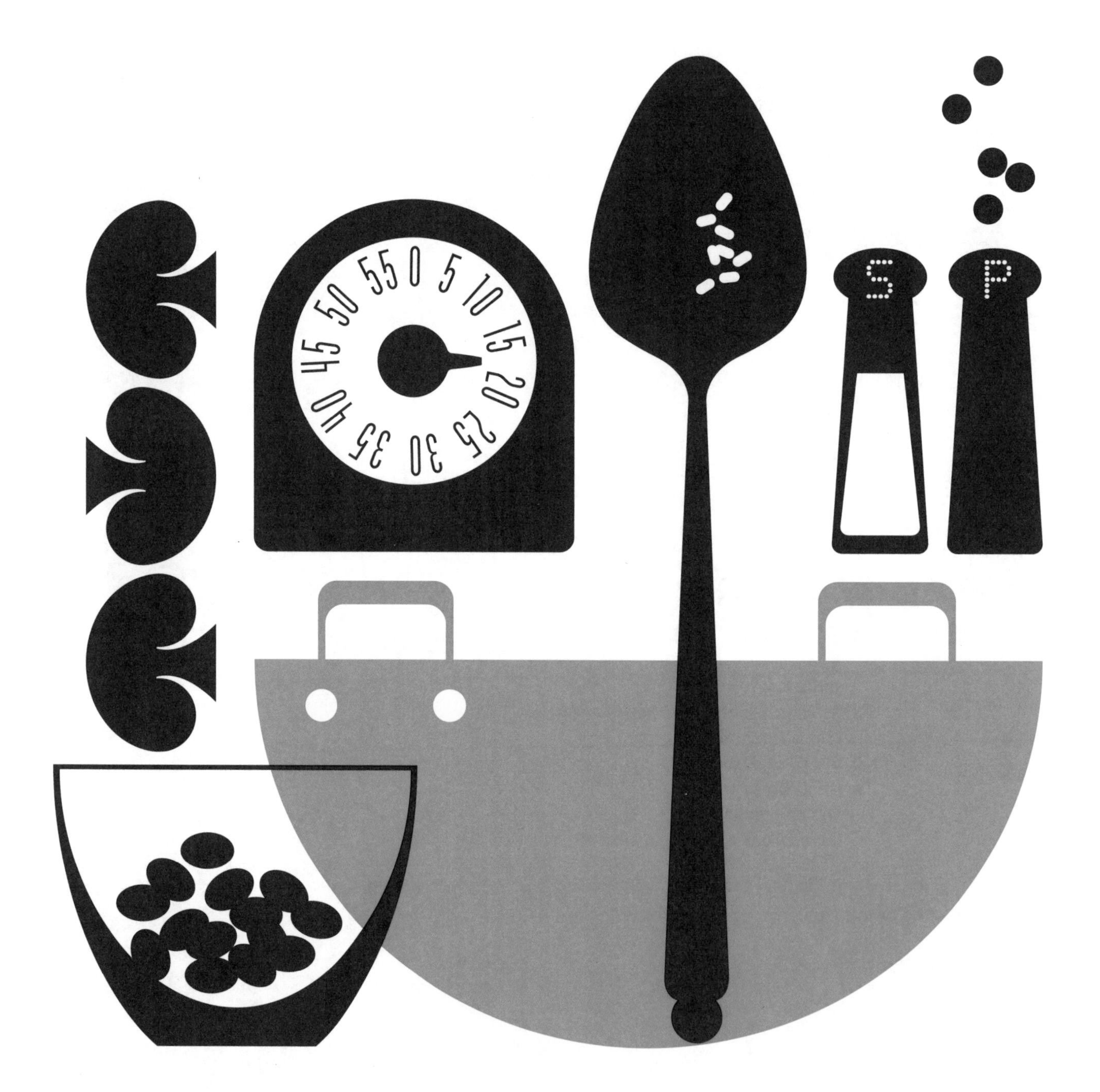
0 5 10 15 20 25 30 35 40 45 50 55
S
P

# chapter 5

## vegetarian meals

We have included a great variety of suggestions for vegetarian cooking in this section. However, vegetarian options are in no way confined to this section. There are many more vegetarian and vegan recipes throughout the book — just look for the vegetarian and vegan icons pictured below. As for what *vegetarian* means, in this book vegetarian suggestions do not include fish, shellfish, or any other meat, but they may include eggs and often feature cheese, yogurt, or milk. Vegan suggestions do not use eggs, honey, or dairy of any sort. Please note that many of our pastas are marked vegetarian; although most pasta has egg in it, eggless brands are available.

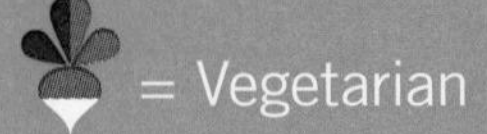 = Vegetarian 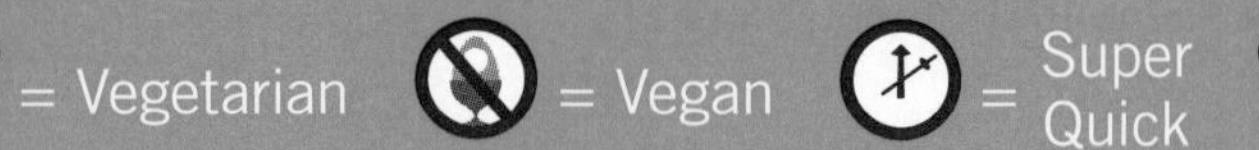 = Vegan 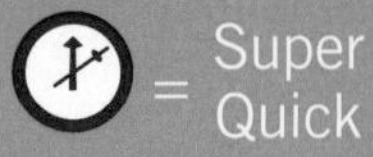 = Super Quick 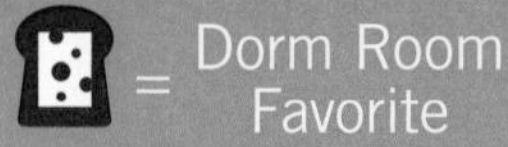 = Dorm Room Favorite

# slow-cooker vegetable stew

MAKES 6 TO 8 SERVINGS

A slow cooker is a wonderful addition to the college student's kitchen. Load it up with ingredients in the morning and return to a warm dinner at the end of your busy day.

- **1 cup warm water**
- **½ cup vegetable oil**
- **¼ cup peanut butter (smooth or crunchy)**
- **3 tablespoons low-sodium soy sauce**
- **1 teaspoon salt**
- **1 teaspoon minced garlic**
- **¼ teaspoon freshly ground black pepper**
- **1 (1-pound) package firm tofu, cut into small chunks**
- **2 cups chopped potato**
- **4–6 carrots, peeled and sliced**
- **2 sweet onions, chopped**
- **2 celery stalks, sliced**

1. Combine the water, oil, peanut butter, soy sauce, salt, garlic, and pepper in a bowl. Whisk together until thoroughly blended. Add the tofu, stir well to coat, cover, and marinate in the refrigerator for several hours or overnight.
2. Combine the potato, carrots, onions, and celery with the tofu and its marinade in a slow cooker. Cook on the low setting for 8 to 10 hours, until the vegetables are tender.

NUTRITION PER SERVING

Calories 300 • Fat 21 g • Fiber 4 g • Protein 10 g • Carbohydrates 21 g

# vegetable chili

MAKES 10 SERVINGS

This is a great winter dish. We recommend making this one for a large group of friends, or just making up a large batch over the weekend to freeze for quick meals throughout the week. Try serving it with warm corn bread, corn chips, or rice.

- **Cooking spray**
- **1 yellow onion, diced**
- **2 green bell peppers, seeded and diced**
- **2 (14.5-ounce) cans stewed whole tomatoes**
- **2 (15-ounce) cans black beans**
- **1 (16-ounce) can whole-kernel corn**
- **1 (15-ounce) can kidney beans**
- **½ tablespoon chili powder**
- **1 teaspoon cayenne pepper**
- **½ teaspoon cinnamon**
- **Salt and freshly ground black pepper**
- **2 tomatoes, diced**
- **2 cups shredded low-fat cheddar cheese (optional)**

1. Spray a large pot with cooking spray and heat over medium heat. Add the onion and green peppers and sauté until they just begin to brown.
2. Add all of the canned ingredients, including the liquid from the cans, as well as the chili powder, cayenne, and cinnamon. Bring to a boil, reduce heat, and simmer for at least 30 minutes, or until the mixture reaches desired consistency. Season to taste with salt and pepper.
3. Ladle into bowls, topping with diced tomatoes and cheese, if using.

NUTRITION PER SERVING

Calories 150 • Fat 0.5 g • Fiber 8 g • Protein 8 g • Carbohydrates 31 g

# african groundnut stew

MAKES 8 SERVINGS

This recipe takes some time to cook, but it's easy to pull together and makes a lot, so you can cook one night and enjoy several meals for your efforts.

**2 tablespoons vegetable oil**
**1 onion, diced**
**3 garlic cloves, minced**
**2 sweet potatoes, peeled and cut into 1-inch cubes**
**1 cup rice**
**8 cups vegetable broth**
**⅓ cup peanut butter (smooth or crunchy)**
**1 (15-ounce) can chickpeas, rinsed and drained**
**3 cups salsa**
**1 cup diced zucchini**
**½ teaspoon cumin**
**1 teaspoon dried thyme**
**Salt and freshly ground black pepper**

1. Heat the oil in a large stockpot over medium heat. Add the onion, garlic, and sweet potatoes and sauté 7 to 10 minutes, until the sweet potatoes are tender.
2. Add the rice and vegetable broth to the pot. Bring to a boil, reduce heat, and simmer, covered, 20 to 30 minutes, until the rice is tender.
3. Add the peanut butter, chickpeas, salsa, zucchini, cumin, thyme, and salt and pepper; cook over low heat until the zucchini is soft.

NUTRITION PER SERVING

Calories 400 • Fat 12 g • Fiber 13 g • Protein 16 g • Carbohydrates 59 g

# teriyaki couscous

MAKES 4 SERVINGS

If you don't have all of the vegetables listed on hand, just use what you have.

- **1 tablespoon extra-virgin olive oil**
- **½ cup chopped onion**
- **½ cup chopped green bell pepper**
- **½ cup chopped mushrooms**
- **½ cup chopped eggplant**
- **3 teaspoons freshly grated ginger**
- **2 tablespoons low-sodium soy sauce**
- **1 teaspoon white vinegar**
- **3 cups cooked couscous**

1. Heat the oil in a large skillet over medium heat. Add the vegetables, 2 teaspoons of the ginger, and 1 tablespoon of the soy sauce. Sauté 7 to 10 minutes, until the vegetables are tender and beginning to turn golden.
2. Add the remaining soy sauce and ginger, vinegar, and couscous. Cook for 1 minute over high heat, stirring often to blend the ingredients.

NUTRITION PER SERVING

Calories 190 • Fat 4 g • Fiber 3 g • Protein 6 g • Carbohydrates 33 g

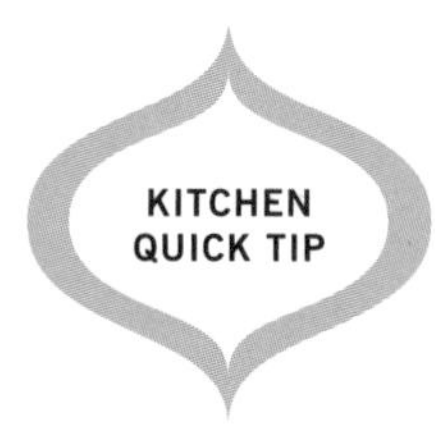


## vitamin c

Did you know that red and green bell peppers have more vitamin C than oranges do? Raw green bells have about twice as much as oranges, while red bells have four times as much!

# curried potatoes

MAKES 4 SERVINGS

The curry powder and soy sauce give these potatoes a pleasant sweet/salty flavor.

**1½ tablespoons extra-virgin olive oil**
**2 large potatoes, peeled and sliced**
**1 small onion, chopped**
**1 tablespoon curry powder**
**1 teaspoon freshly grated ginger**
**½ teaspoon salt**
**1 teaspoon sugar**
**3 tablespoons low-sodium soy sauce**

1. Heat the oil in a large skillet over medium heat. Add the potatoes and cook, stirring often, for 15 minutes or until browned.

2. Add the onion, curry, and ginger to the skillet. Cook for 1 minute, stirring. Add the salt, sugar, and soy sauce. Cook for another 5 minutes, stirring often, until the potatoes are completely tender. Add a few tablespoons of water if the pan dries out before the potatoes are cooked.

NUTRITION PER SERVING
Calories 210 • Fat 6 g • Fiber 4 g • Protein 5 g • Carbohydrates 37 g

# black beans and onions

MAKES 4 SERVINGS

This recipe takes practically no time. It's good on its own (hot or cold) or as a topping for brown rice. If you're planning on having this as your main dish, you might want to make a bit more than what is called for here.

**1 teaspoon butter**
**1 medium onion, chopped**
**1 (15-ounce) can black beans, rinsed and drained**
**Salt and freshly ground black pepper**

1. Melt the butter in a skillet over medium heat. Add the onion and sauté for 5 minutes. The onion should stay crisp, but not brown.
2. Add the beans and cook for 3 to 4 minutes longer, until the onion is translucent. Season with salt and pepper to taste.

NUTRITION PER SERVING
Calories 80 • Fat 1 g • Fiber 5 g • Protein 4 g • Carbohydrates 17 g

# hoppin' john

MAKES 2 SERVINGS

Hoppin' John is traditionally served in the South as a good-luck dish on New Year's Day. You can add leftover chicken or pork or grated cheese to the dish if you desire. It's inexpensive and delicious southern comfort food!

**1 (16-ounce) can black-eyed peas, rinsed and drained**
**2 cups cooked brown rice**
**2 tablespoons hot pepper sauce (or to taste)**

Combine all ingredients in a saucepan and heat on a stovetop, stirring often, until hot. You can also combine the ingredients in a microwave-safe bowl, cover, and microwave for about 3 minutes or until heated through. Serve immediately.

NUTRITION PER SERVING
Calories 350 • Fat 2 g • Fiber 11 g • Protein 16 g • Carbohydrates 73 g

# red beans and rice

MAKES 4 SERVINGS

Serve these spicy beans over hot cooked rice.

**1 teaspoon butter**
**1 small yellow onion, chopped**
**½ green bell pepper, seeded and chopped**
**1 celery stalk, chopped**
**2 (15-ounce) cans kidney beans, rinsed and drained**
**2 garlic cloves, minced**
**½ teaspoon dried oregano**
**½ cup tomato sauce**
**1 tablespoon hot sauce**
**2 tablespoons Worcestershire sauce**
**Salt and freshly ground black pepper**

1. Melt the butter in a large skillet over medium heat. Add the onion and sauté until it becomes translucent, about 3 minutes.
2. Add the green pepper, celery, beans, garlic, oregano, tomato sauce, hot sauce, and Worcestershire. Simmer over low heat for 10 minutes. Season to taste with salt and pepper and serve immediately.

NUTRITION PER SERVING

Calories 220 • Fat 2 g • Fiber 13 g • Protein 12 g • Carbohydrates 41 g

# caramelized onion orzo

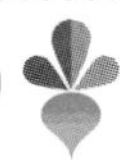

MAKES 4 SERVINGS

Orzo is a small, delicate pasta that looks a lot like rice. You will find it in the pasta section of your local supermarket.

**1 (8-ounce) package orzo**
**1 tablespoon butter**
**3 tablespoons packed brown sugar**
**2 medium onions, chopped**

1. Cook the orzo according to the package directions. Drain.
2. Melt the butter and sugar in a skillet over medium heat. Add the onions and sauté until brown, about 12 minutes.
3. Combine the onion mixture with the orzo. Serve warm.

NUTRITION PER SERVING

Calories 290 • Fat 3.5 g • Fiber 3 g • Protein 8 g • Carbohydrates 58 g

# lemony tofu over greens

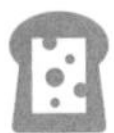

MAKES 4 SERVINGS

Fresh and light yet filling.

**1 (1-pound) package extra-firm tofu**
**¼ cup low-sodium soy sauce**
**3 tablespoons lemon juice**
**3 scallions, sliced**
**Spring-mix salad greens (1 large handful per person)**

1. Cut the tofu in half horizontally. Place the halves between paper towels and blot dry. Cut tofu into bite-size cubes and place in a single layer in a casserole dish or plastic container.

2. Mix together the soy sauce and lemon juice in a small bowl. Pour over the tofu and sprinkle the scallions over the top. Marinate in the refrigerator for 1 hour before serving over salad greens.

NUTRITION PER SERVING

Calories 130 • Fat 6 g • Fiber 2 g • Protein 13 g • Carbohydrates 6 g

# ginger-soy tofu with rice

MAKES 4 SERVINGS

Serve with a salad tossed with an Asian dressing for a lighter dinner.

**1 tablespoon extra-virgin olive oil**
**1 (1-pound) package firm tofu, sliced into thin strips**
**⅓ cup low-sodium soy sauce**
**1 teaspoon freshly grated ginger**
**3 cups hot cooked rice (about 1½ cups uncooked)**

1. Heat the oil in a large skillet over medium heat. Add the tofu and sauté for 5 minutes.
2. Combine the soy sauce and ginger in a small bowl.
3. Add half of the soy sauce mixture to the skillet. Reduce the heat to low and cook the tofu for 2 minutes.
4. Flip the strips of tofu and add the remaining half of the soy sauce mixture. Cook for 5 minutes longer. Serve over hot cooked rice.

NUTRITION PER SERVING

Calories 410 • Fat 10 g • Fiber 2 g • Protein 18 g • Carbohydrates 60 g

# meg's thai tofu

MAKES 4 SERVINGS

Peanut butter is the secret ingredient in this complete tofu dinner.

- Cooking spray
- 2 cups brown rice
- ½ cup natural peanut butter
- ¼ cup water
- ¼ cup low-sodium soy sauce
- 2 tablespoons rice vinegar, or whatever vinegar you have
- 2 garlic cloves, minced, or 1 tablespoon garlic powder
- 1 (1-pound) package extra-firm tofu, cut into cubes
- 1 (16-ounce) package frozen stir-fry vegetable mix
- Sesame seeds, chopped peanuts, or chopped scallions (optional, for garnish)

1. Preheat the oven to 350°F. Coat a baking dish with cooking spray.
2. Cook the rice according to the package directions.
3. While the rice is cooking, combine the peanut butter, water, soy sauce, vinegar, and garlic in a saucepan. Stir over low heat until smooth and creamy.
4. Add the tofu to the sauce and pour into the prepared baking dish. Bake the tofu for 20 minutes.
5. While the tofu is baking, cook the frozen vegetables according to the package directions.
6. Remove the tofu from the oven, stir in the hot vegetables, and serve the mixture over hot rice. Top with sesame seeds, chopped peanuts, and/or scallions, if using.

NUTRITION PER SERVING

Calories 680 • Fat 25 g • Fiber 8 g • Protein 29 g • Carbohydrates 87 g

# garlic green beans with tofu

MAKES 4 SERVINGS

This recipe makes four servings as a side dish and two servings as a main dish.

**1 pound green beans**
**2 tablespoons vegetable oil**
**4 garlic cloves, minced**
**½ (1-pound) package firm tofu, cut into bite-size pieces**
**Salt and freshly ground black pepper**

1. Rinse the beans and snip off their ends.
2. Heat the oil in a wok or nonstick skillet over medium heat. Add the beans and garlic and stir-fry for 5 minutes.
3. Add the tofu and stir-fry for 5 minutes longer. Season to taste with salt and pepper.

NUTRITION PER SERVING
Calories 150 • Fat 10 g • Fiber 3 g • Protein 7 g • Carbohydrates 8 g

## 6 quick ideas for steamed vegetables

- Dust with your favorite herbs and spices.
- Top with Parmesan.
- Sprinkle with lemon juice and pepper.
- Drizzle with your favorite salad dressing.
- Marinate in a touch of white wine and serve over rice.
- Toss in with some eggs and make an omelet.

# tofu and broccoli stir-fry

MAKES 2 SERVINGS

This recipe includes a great peanut sauce, but if you're not one for peanut butter, please don't skip over the whole recipe — try a splash of soy sauce instead. Both variations are delicious over brown or white rice.

**1 tablespoon peanut butter**
**1 tablespoon hot water**
**1 tablespoon cider vinegar**
**1 tablespoon low-sodium soy sauce**
**2 teaspoons canola oil**
**3 cups chopped broccoli**
**2 garlic cloves, minced**
**½ (1-pound) package firm tofu, cut into small cubes**

1. Stir together the peanut butter, hot water, vinegar, and soy sauce in a small bowl. If it is difficult to mix, microwave on high for 10 seconds to soften the peanut butter.
2. Heat the oil in a wok or large nonstick skillet over high heat. Add the broccoli and garlic and stir-fry for 5 minutes.
3. Add the tofu and stir-fry for 5 minutes longer. Remove from the heat.
4. Pour the sauce over the tofu and broccoli and mix well.

NUTRITION PER SERVING

Calories 220 • Fat 14 g • Fiber 10 g • Protein 16 g • Carbohydrates 13 g

# sesame noodles

MAKES 4 SERVINGS

This can be an incredibly fast recipe if you have leftover pasta in the fridge and don't need to cook it. This is one pasta dish that tastes much better served cold.

**8 ounces spaghetti**
**¼ cup peanut butter**
**2 teaspoons sesame oil**
**½ teaspoon cider vinegar**
**1 tablespoon chopped scallions (optional)**

1. Cook the pasta according to the package directions.
2. Combine the peanut butter, sesame oil, and vinegar in a small microwave-safe bowl. Microwave on high for 30 seconds, until the peanut butter begins to melt. Mix well. (If you don't have a microwave, you can also do this in a skillet over low heat.)
3. Blend the peanut butter mixture into the pasta. Add the scallions, if using. Refrigerate and serve cold.

NUTRITION PER SERVING
Calories 320 • Fat 11 g • Fiber 3 g • Protein 11 g • Carbohydrates 45 g

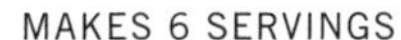

# spinach pie

MAKES 6 SERVINGS

This dish can satisfy a quiche craving without crushing a diet.

- **1 (10-ounce) package frozen spinach**
- **1 cup fat-free cottage cheese**
- **3 eggs, beaten**
- **¼ cup grated Parmesan cheese**
- **1 small onion, finely chopped**
- **1 teaspoon garlic salt**
- **1 teaspoon freshly ground pepper**
- **1 teaspoon Tabasco sauce**
- **½ teaspoon ground nutmeg**
- **¼ cup shredded low-fat Swiss cheese**

1. Preheat the oven to 350°F.
2. Cook the spinach according to the package directions. When it's cool enough to touch, squeeze out as much liquid as you can from the leaves.
3. Combine the spinach, cottage cheese, eggs, Parmesan, onion, garlic salt, pepper, Tabasco, and nutmeg in a large bowl, and mix well.
4. Spread the mixture in a pie plate, and top with the Swiss cheese. Bake for 40 to 50 minutes, or until the top is light brown and a knife inserted into the middle comes out clean. Serve warm.

NUTRITION PER SERVING

Calories 110 • Fat 4 g • Fiber 2 g • Protein 11 g • Carbohydrates 7 g

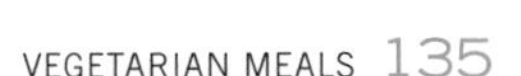

# anna's veggie lasagna

MAKES 8 SERVINGS

This one is highly recommended for large groups or potlucks. Everyone loves lasagna.

**1 (16-ounce) package lasagna noodles**
**½ tablespoon extra-virgin olive oil**
**1 large yellow onion, chopped**
**2 carrots, peeled and grated**
**1 medium zucchini, chopped**
**4 ounces white mushrooms, wiped clean and chopped**
**3 lightly packed cups fresh spinach**
**1 (16-ounce) container fat-free cottage cheese**
**Salt and freshly ground black pepper**
**5 cups tomato sauce**
**1½ cups shredded low-fat mozzarella cheese**

1. Preheat the oven to 350°F.
2. Bring a large pot of water to a boil. Salt the water and add the noodles; cook until they are pliable but only half cooked, 4 to 5 minutes. Remove the noodles from the water and place them in a bowl of cold water to stop the cooking.
3. Heat the oil in a large skillet over medium heat. Add the onion, carrots, and zucchini and sauté until the onion is translucent, about 3 minutes. Add the mushrooms and continue to sauté until they begin to soften, about 3 minutes. Add the spinach and cook about 3 minutes longer, until it wilts and shrinks.
4. Add the cottage cheese and cook for 5 to 7 minutes, until the flavors are well mixed. Season to taste with salt and pepper. Remove from the heat and drain any excess liquid from the pan.
5. Spread a thin layer of tomato sauce in a large lasagna pan. Place a layer of noodles on top of it, followed by a layer of cheese and then a layer of the sautéed vegetables. Repeat until the dish is almost full. Top with a layer of noodles covered with a layer of cheese. Cover with aluminum foil and bake for 40 minutes.

NUTRITION PER SERVING

Calories 370 • Fat 6 g • Fiber 5 g • Protein 22 g • Carbohydrates 60 g

# spinach calzone

MAKES 2 SERVINGS

This calzone is very tasty, can be created with very few supplies, and provides a full serving of vegetables. Though it's easiest to prepare on a George Foreman Grill, you could also grill it in a skillet.

**1 cup marinara sauce**
**1 cup shredded mozzarella cheese**
**1 cup chopped spinach (frozen is fine; thaw and squeeze the water from it)**
**2 pita rounds**

1. Preheat a George Foreman Grill.
2. Mix the sauce and cheese together in a small bowl. Stir in the spinach.
3. Cut the pita rounds in half and open the pockets. Stuff each half with the spinach mixture. Place the stuffed pitas in the George Foreman Grill so that the open side of the pita faces the hinges of the grill (this prevents the stuffing from falling out). Close the grill and cook for 3 minutes, or until heated through and the cheese is melted. Enjoy!

NUTRITION PER SERVING

Calories 270 • Fat 11 g • Fiber 4 g • Protein 20 g • Carbohydrates 25 g

# eggplant parmesan

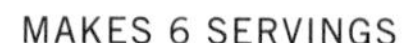

MAKES 6 SERVINGS

If you have fresh basil, use it in this recipe.

**½ cup breadcrumbs**
**1 tablespoon dried oregano**
**1 tablespoon dried basil**
**5 tablespoons extra-virgin olive oil**
**1 medium eggplant, cut into ½-inch slices**
**1 garlic clove, minced**
**2½ cups crushed tomatoes (canned tomatoes are fine)**
**Salt and freshly ground black pepper**
**⅓ (1-pound) block of mozzarella cheese (or enough to cover the dish), thinly sliced**
**¼ cup grated Parmesan cheese**

1. Preheat the oven to 350°F.
2. Combine the breadcrumbs, oregano, and basil in a shallow dish.
3. Heat most of the oil (reserving about 1 teaspoon) in a skillet over medium heat. Dip each slice of eggplant into the breadcrumbs, coating both sides, and drop into the skillet. Cook for about 2 minutes per side, or until golden brown.
4. Place the eggplant in a single layer in an ungreased baking dish.
5. Heat the reserved teaspoon of oil in a saucepan over medium heat. Add the garlic and sauté for 1 minute, then add the tomatoes and salt and pepper to taste. Simmer for 5 minutes to blend the flavors.
6. Pour the tomato sauce over the eggplant slices. Top with mozzarella and sprinkle Parmesan evenly over the dish.
7. Bake for 30 minutes. Remove from the oven and cool for 10 minutes before serving.

NUTRITION PER SERVING

Calories 290 • Fat 19 g • Fiber 6 g • Protein 11 g • Carbohydrates 20 g

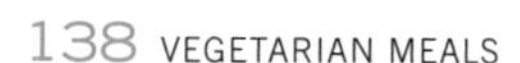

# two-bean tamale pie

MAKES 4 SERVINGS

A tasty all-in-one meal.

- **Cooking spray**
- **1 tablespoon vegetable oil**
- **1 green bell pepper, seeded and chopped**
- **1 onion, chopped**
- **2 garlic cloves, minced**
- **1 (15-ounce) can kidney beans, rinsed, drained, and slightly mashed**
- **1 (15-ounce) can pinto beans, rinsed, drained, and slightly mashed**
- **1 (16-ounce) can whole-kernel corn, drained, or 1 cup frozen or fresh corn kernels**
- **6 ounces vegetable juice**
- **1 (4-ounce) can diced green chiles**
- **1 teaspoon chili powder**
- **½ teaspoon ground cumin**
- **1 (8.5- to 10-ounce) package corn bread mix**
- **½ cup shredded cheddar cheese**
- **Chopped fresh cilantro or parsley**

1. Preheat the oven to 400°F. Coat a 2-quart baking dish with cooking spray.
2. Heat the oil in a large skillet over medium heat. Add the green pepper, onion, and garlic and sauté 3 to 5 minutes, until tender. Stir in the beans, corn, vegetable juice, chiles, chili powder, and cumin and continue to cook until the mixture is heated through.
3. Spoon the bean mixture into the prepared baking dish.
4. Prepare the corn bread batter according to the package directions. Stir in the cheese and a small handful of cilantro or parsley. Spoon the corn bread batter on top of the bean mixture in an even layer. Bake uncovered for 25 to 35 minutes, until the corn bread is cooked through and golden brown on top.

NUTRITION PER SERVING

Calories 910 • Fat 49 g • Fiber 18 g • Protein 24 g • Carbohydrates 93 g

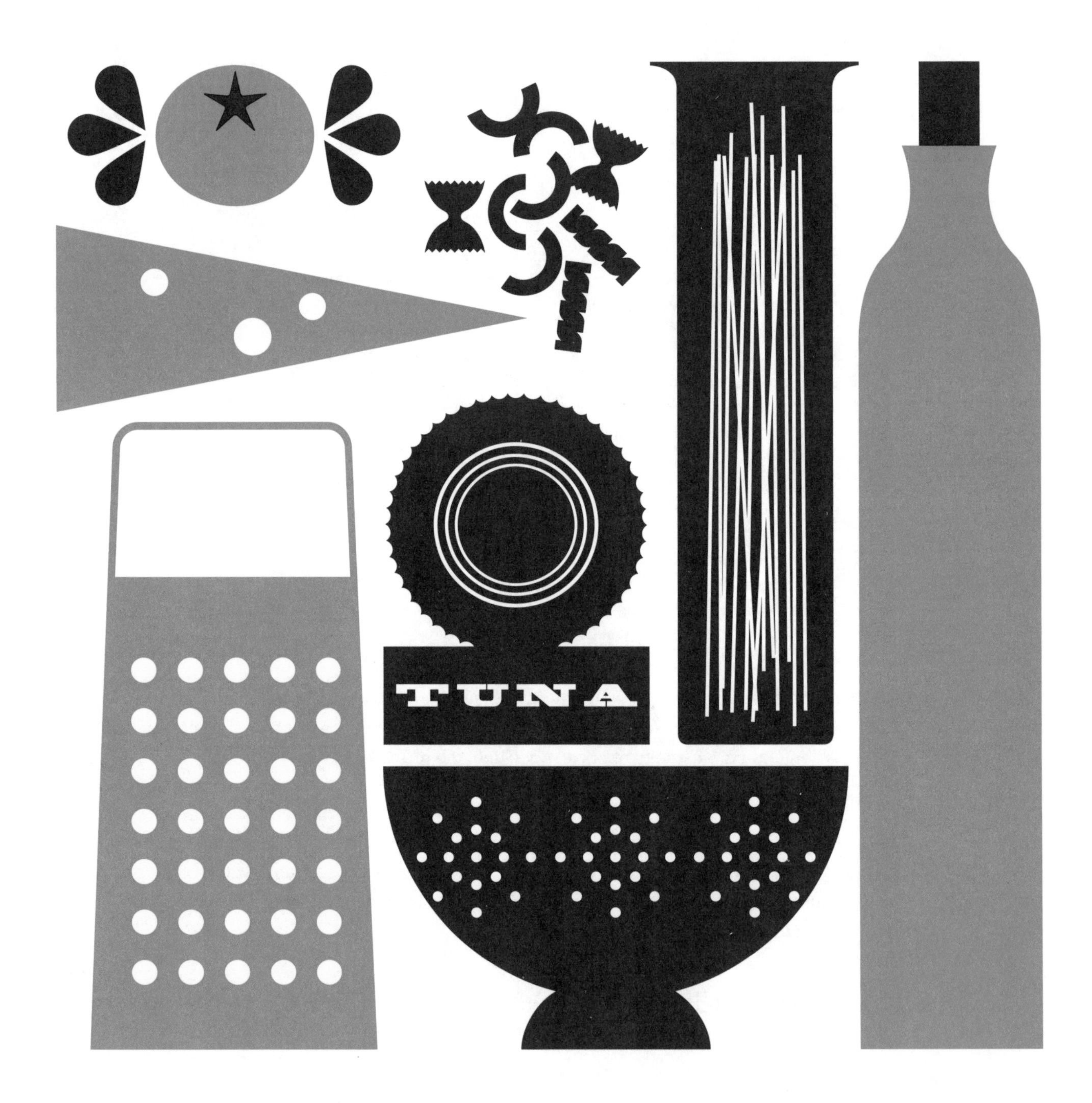
TUNA

# chapter 6

## pasta, pasta & more pasta

Pasta has acquired a reputation as a last-resort lifesaver for college students cooking on their own. While spaghetti with tomato sauce and microwave macaroni and cheese are worthwhile dishes for any first-time cook, we hope to provide a wider range of options. Feel free to mix and match pasta shapes with sauces.

We've listed some great pasta sauces in this chapter. However, to figure out the nutritional information of a serving of sauce over a serving-size portion of pasta (usually 2 ounces), you'll need to know the nutritional breakdown for plain pasta. Here's a comparison of 2 ounces of enriched pasta versus 2 ounces of whole-wheat pasta:

| ENRICHED PASTA | WHOLE-WHEAT PASTA |
|---|---|
| Calories 210 | Calories 180 |
| Fat 1 g | Fat 2 g |
| Carbohydrates 42 g | Carbohydrates 41 g |
| Protein 7 g | Protein 7 g |
| Cholesterol 0 g | Cholesterol 0 g |
| Fiber 2 g | Fiber 6 g |

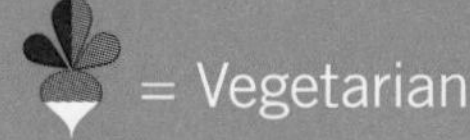

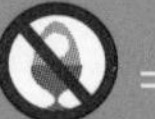
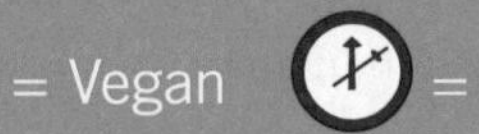

= Super Quick
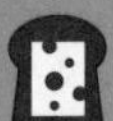
= Dorm Room Favorite

## sweet red pepper sauce

MAKES 4 SERVINGS

**1 teaspoon extra-virgin olive oil**
**2 red bell peppers, seeded and chopped**
**2 carrots, peeled and chopped**
**2 medium tomatoes, chopped**
**1 garlic clove, minced**
**1 pear, peeled and sliced**
**1 teaspoon salt**
**½ teaspoon freshly ground black pepper**
**1 teaspoon dried basil**

1. Heat the oil in a skillet over medium heat. Add the red peppers and carrots and sauté until soft, about 10 minutes.
2. Add the tomatoes, garlic, pear, salt, pepper, and basil to the skillet. Reduce the heat and simmer for about 30 minutes.
3. Purée the vegetable mixture in a blender. Serve over hot pasta.

NUTRITION PER SERVING
Calories 90 • Fat 1.5 g • Fiber 5 g • Protein 2 g • Carbohydrates 19 g

## tomato-basil sauce

MAKES 4 SERVINGS

**1 teaspoon extra-virgin olive oil**
**2 garlic cloves, minced**
**Salt and freshly ground black pepper**
**1 (15-ounce) can diced tomatoes, drained**
**1 tablespoon chopped fresh basil**

1. Heat the oil in a saucepan over medium heat. Add the garlic and sauté for about 1 minute, or until lightly browned. Season with salt and pepper.
2. Add the tomatoes and cook for 10 minutes, stirring often. Add the basil and stir well. Serve over hot pasta.

NUTRITION PER SERVING
Calories 40 • Fat 1 g • Fiber 1 g • Protein 1 g • Carbohydrates 5 g

# basic tomato sauce

MAKES 4 SERVINGS

This recipe is far better than the store-bought stuff and will save you money in the long run. For a little variety, you can add almost any vegetable from your refrigerator. Serve it over any pasta in your cupboard — we prefer spaghetti.

**1 teaspoon extra-virgin olive oil**
**2 garlic cloves, minced**
**1 (20-ounce) can tomato sauce**
**1 (6-ounce) can tomato paste**
**¼ teaspoon salt**
**¼ teaspoon freshly ground black pepper**
**1 teaspoon dried basil**
**1 teaspoon dried oregano**

1. Heat the oil in a saucepan over medium heat. Add the garlic and sauté for about 1 minute, until the garlic is lightly browned.
2. Add the tomato sauce and paste, salt, pepper, basil, and oregano, and mix well. Bring to a boil, then reduce heat and simmer for 5 minutes.
3. Serve immediately over hot pasta, or cool and ladle into containers for refrigeration or freezing.

NUTRITION PER SERVING
Calories 90 • Fat 1.5 g • Fiber 4 g • Protein 5 g • Carbohydrates 16 g

## for a little variety

To make your tomato sauce a little more exciting, we recommend sautéing vegetables along with the garlic before adding the tomato sauce. If you want to add meat, make sure that it's cooked well before adding it to your sauce. Here are some suggestions for tomato sauce additions:

- Zucchini and yellow squash
- Mushrooms
- Spinach
- Onion
- Broccoli
- Ground beef or turkey

# mushroom sauce

MAKES 3 SERVINGS

In addition to being a delicious pasta sauce, the creamy mushrooms are wonderful with white or brown rice or even spooned over crusty toast for a really quick meal.

**3 tablespoons butter**
**12 ounces mushrooms, wiped clean and sliced**
**⅓ cup white wine**
**1½ cups all-purpose flour**
**1¼ cups low-fat milk**
**¼ teaspoon salt**
**¼ teaspoon freshly ground black pepper**

1. Melt the butter in a large skillet over medium heat. Add the mushrooms and sauté 6 to 8 minutes, until they are soft and have released their liquid. Add the wine, increase the heat to high, and cook until the wine has been absorbed.
2. Reduce the heat to low. Add the flour, stirring to coat the mushrooms. Slowly pour in the milk and cook, stirring constantly, until the sauce thickens. Season with salt and pepper. Serve over hot pasta.

NUTRITION PER SERVING
Calories 410 • Fat 13 g • Fiber 3 g • Protein 14 g • Carbohydrates 57 g

# emily's garlic-mushroom sauce

MAKES 2 SERVINGS

Serve this recipe over hot bow-tie pasta. A splash of sherry added to the mushrooms would be great.

**1 teaspoon butter**
**6 ounces mushrooms, wiped clean and sliced**
**1 garlic clove, minced**
**Pinch of salt**
**2 tablespoons grated Parmesan cheese**

1. Melt the butter in a skillet over medium heat. Add the mushrooms and garlic and sauté until the mushrooms are soft and have released their liquid, about 8 minutes. Add the salt.
2. Spoon the mushrooms over hot pasta and sprinkle with Parmesan.

NUTRITION PER SERVING

Calories 60 • Fat 4 g • Fiber 0 g • Protein 4 g • Carbohydrates 4 g

# spinach-ricotta sauce

MAKES 4 SERVINGS

**2 teaspoons extra-virgin olive oil**
**1 medium onion, chopped**
**2 garlic cloves, minced**
**1 cup cooked spinach**
**1 cup nonfat ricotta cheese**
**1 large tomato, chopped**
**¼ teaspoon freshly ground black pepper**
**Salt**
**¼ cup grated Parmesan cheese**

1. Heat the oil in a large skillet over medium heat. Add the onion and garlic and sauté 4 to 6 minutes, until the onion is translucent.
2. Add the spinach, ricotta, tomato, and pepper. Mix thoroughly; season with salt to taste. Add the Parmesan; mix well. Serve over hot pasta.

NUTRITION PER SERVING

Calories 110 • Fat 4 g • Fiber 1 g • Protein 11 g • Carbohydrates 9 g

# macaroni and cheese

MAKES 4 SERVINGS

When you're craving macaroni and cheese, try this yogurt-lightened version instead of the orange boxed stuff.

- **1¾ cups macaroni**
- **1 cup shredded low-fat cheddar cheese**
- **¼ cup nonfat plain yogurt**
- **2 teaspoons butter**
- **½ tablespoon Dijon mustard**
- **Salt and freshly ground black pepper**

1. Bring a large pot of water to a boil. Salt the water and add the macaroni; cook until tender, about 8 minutes.
2. While the pasta is cooking, mix together the cheese and yogurt.
3. When the pasta is done, drain and set aside. Put the pot back on the stove over medium heat and add the butter. When the butter is melted, stir in the mustard and season with salt and pepper. Add the cooked macaroni, tossing to coat. Mix in the cheese and yogurt. Continue to cook, stirring constantly, until the cheese is melted.

NUTRITION PER SERVING

Calories 240 • Fat 4.5 g • Fiber 1 g • Protein 14 g • Carbohydrates 36 g

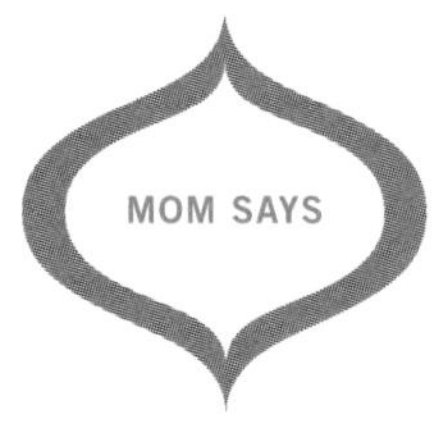


Always add a tablespoon or two of salt to your pasta water. It brings out the flavor of the pasta and helps the sauce adhere.

# fettuccine alfredo

MAKES 4 SERVINGS

Cottage cheese and Parmesan give this fettuccine the luscious creaminess usually provided by lots of butter and heavy cream.

**8 ounces fettuccine**
**1 cup fat-free cottage cheese**
**⅓ cup grated Parmesan cheese**
**¼ cup skim milk**
**Salt and freshly ground black pepper**
**1 cup cooked vegetables (try carrots, broccoli, mushrooms, or whatever else you have)**

1. Bring a large pot of water to a boil. Salt the water and add the fettuccine; cook until tender, about 10 minutes. Drain. Return the pasta to the pot and set aside.
2. While the pasta is cooking, purée the cottage cheese in a blender until it is smooth. Add the Parmesan, milk, and salt and pepper to taste. Blend until smooth.
3. Pour the sauce over the pasta and stir in the vegetables. Cook over medium heat, stirring frequently, for 2 to 3 minutes, or until thoroughly mixed and heated.

NUTRITION PER SERVING

Calories 290 • Fat 3 g • Fiber 3 g • Protein 18 g • Carbohydrates 50 g

# teriyaki salmon over pasta

MAKES 4 SERVINGS

Canned salmon is perfect for this recipe — and it has all the health benefits of fresh salmon.

**8 ounces pasta**
**1 teaspoon extra-virgin olive oil**
**6 medium mushrooms, wiped clean and sliced**
**1 garlic clove, minced**
**1 teaspoon low-sodium soy sauce, or more to taste**
**½ teaspoon freshly grated ginger**
**1 (7.5-ounce) can pink salmon, drained**

1. Bring a large pot of water to a boil. Salt the water and add the pasta; cook according to the package directions. Drain and set aside.
2. Heat the oil in a large skillet over medium heat. Add the mushrooms and garlic and sauté until the mushrooms begin to soften and release their liquid, about 8 minutes. Season with the soy sauce and ginger. Mix well. Increase the heat to medium-high and cook for 3 minutes longer.
3. Mix in the salmon, adding more soy sauce to taste. Add the cooked pasta and stir well. Cook for 2 minutes longer, stirring constantly. Serve hot.

NUTRITION PER SERVING

Calories 310 • Fat 6 g • Fiber 2 g • Protein 19 g • Carbohydrates 44 g

# ramen noodle stir-fry

MAKES 2 SERVINGS

Ramen noodles are fast, cheap, and versatile. Many brands are high in fat, so be sure to buy the low-fat baked noodles. You can also substitute four ounces of any type of pasta or rice, but the dish will take longer to prepare.

**1 package baked ramen noodles (any flavor — you won't be using the seasoning packet)**
**1 teaspoon extra-virgin olive oil**
**¼ cup chopped green bell pepper**
**¼ cup chopped red bell pepper**
**¼ cup chopped onion**
**1 garlic clove, minced**
**1 teaspoon hot sauce**
**Dried oregano**
**Cayenne pepper**

1. Bring a pot of water to a boil. Salt the water and add the noodles; cook until tender, about 3 minutes.

2. Heat the oil in a large skillet over medium heat. Add the bell peppers, onion, and garlic, and sauté until the vegetables are tender. Add the hot sauce and season with oregano and cayenne. Simmer for 5 minutes.

3. Add the noodles to the skillet and cook for about 1 minute, or until thoroughly mixed and heated through.

NUTRITION PER SERVING

Calories 300 • Fat 12 g • Fiber 2 g • Protein 6 g • Carbohydrates 42 g

# thai-inspired beef and pasta

MAKES 2 SERVINGS

The soy sauce marinade is a great change of pace from a traditional pasta sauce.

**3 tablespoons lime juice**
**3 tablespoons low-sodium soy sauce**
**3 tablespoons vegetable oil**
**2 tablespoons packed brown sugar**
**¼ teaspoon garlic powder**
**¼ teaspoon ground ginger**
**¼ teaspoon curry powder**
**1 (6-ounce) eye-round steak**
**1 cup uncooked elbow macaroni**
**¼ cup thinly sliced onions**
**1 garlic clove, minced**
**1 cup thinly sliced red bell pepper**
**⅓ cup sesame seeds**
**¼ cup crumbled feta cheese**

1. Mix together the lime juice, soy sauce, oil, sugar, garlic powder, ginger, and curry powder in a small bowl. Place the beef in a ziplock bag. Pour half of the marinade into the bag. Squeeze out any air from the bag and seal it. Place in the refrigerator for at least an hour or overnight (the longer it sits, the better the flavor). If you're letting the beef marinate overnight, cover the small bowl with the remaining marinade and refrigerate.

2. When you're ready to eat, bring a pot of water to a boil. Salt the water and add the macaroni; cook 8 to 10 minutes, or until tender. Drain and set aside.

3. While the macaroni is cooking, remove the beef from the ziplock bag and discard the marinade in the bag. Cut the beef into thin strips. Sauté the meat in a large skillet over medium heat until cooked through. Remove the beef from the skillet and set aside.

4. Pour the reserved marinade into the same skillet. Add the onions, garlic, red pepper, and sesame seeds, and sauté until the vegetables are tender. Stir in the browned beef and cooked pasta. Sprinkle with feta and serve.

NUTRITION PER SERVING

Calories 790 • Fat 44 g • Fiber 5 g • Protein 32 g • Carbohydrates 68 g

# creamy mushroom-asparagus pasta

MAKES 4 SERVINGS

If you're hoping to impress, this is the dish to make.

**8 ounces penne**
**14 asparagus stalks, trimmed and cut to 1½-inch lengths**
**2 teaspoons extra-virgin olive oil**
**⅔ cup finely chopped onion**
**10 mushrooms, wiped clean and quartered**
**1 cup sliced ham, cut to approximately the same width and length as the asparagus**
**1 cup light cream, or half-and-half**
**Salt and freshly ground black pepper**

1. Bring a large pot of water to a boil. Salt the water and add the pasta; cook according to the package directions. Drain and set aside.
2. Place the asparagus in a pot and fill with ¼ to ½ inch of water. Bring to a boil, reduce heat, and steam, covered, until the asparagus is tender, 7 to 10 minutes.
3. Heat the oil in a large skillet over medium heat. Add the onion and sauté until it is translucent. Add the mushrooms and ham, and cook until the mushrooms have released their liquid, about 8 minutes.
4. Add the asparagus to the skillet and pour in the cream. Continue to cook over low heat until the sauce thickens, about 8 minutes. Season to taste with salt and pepper. Pour the sauce over the drained pasta and mix well. Serve immediately.

NUTRITION PER SERVING
Calories 490 • Fat 23 g • Fiber 3 g • Protein 23 g • Carbohydrates 49 g

# lemon-asparagus pasta

MAKES 4 TO 6 SERVINGS

This pasta is a perfect choice for when you find tender young asparagus in the spring.

**1½ pounds thin asparagus spears**
**1 pound pasta (campanelle or fusilli works well)**
**¼ cup extra-virgin olive oil**
**¼ cup pine nuts**
**Grated zest of half a lemon (organic if possible, to avoid any pesticides or coatings on the peel)**
**1 teaspoon lemon juice**
**½ teaspoon salt (sea salt is best)**
**½ teaspoon freshly ground black pepper**
**⅓ cup grated Parmesan cheese, plus more for serving**

1. Wash and trim the tough ends from the asparagus, then cut the spears into 1- to 2-inch pieces. Bring a pot of salted water to a boil, add the asparagus, and boil until barely tender. Remove the asparagus from the pot with a slotted spoon (you'll use the water to cook the pasta).
2. Bring the pot of water back to a boil. Add the pasta and cook according to the package directions. Drain and set aside.
3. Combine the cooked asparagus, olive oil, pine nuts, lemon zest, lemon juice, salt, and pepper in a blender or food processor. Blend the ingredients until they form a relatively smooth sauce.
4. Toss the pasta with the asparagus sauce and stir in the Parmesan. Serve immediately, with extra cheese sprinkled over the top.

NUTRITION PER SERVING
Calories 450 • Fat 17 g • Fiber 9 g • Protein 16 g • Carbohydrates 62 g

# easy eggplant pasta

MAKES 4 SERVINGS

You can add to this dish whatever other vegetables or herbs you have on hand.

- 8 ounces pasta (whatever you have on hand)
- 3 tablespoons extra-virgin olive oil
- 1 small onion, chopped
- 2 garlic cloves, minced
- 1 small eggplant, chopped into bite-size pieces
- 1 carrot, peeled and diced
- Salt and freshly ground black pepper
- Pinch of dried basil
- Pinch of dried thyme
- Pinch of dried rosemary
- Handful of fresh parsley, chopped
- 1 (14.5-ounce) can Italian-style diced tomatoes
- Handful of frozen peas
- Shredded mozzarella or grated Parmesan

1. Bring a large pot of water to a boil. Salt the water and add the pasta; cook according to the package directions. Drain and set aside.
2. While the pasta is cooking, heat the olive oil in a large skillet over medium heat. Add the chopped onion and garlic. Sauté, stirring occasionally, about 5 minutes, until the onion is translucent.
3. Add the eggplant, carrot, salt and pepper to taste, dried herbs, and parsley, and sauté for 5 minutes longer, until the carrot is tender.
4. Add the tomatoes with their juice. Bring to a boil, reduce heat, and simmer, covered, for 15 to 20 minutes, until the eggplant is cooked through. Toss in the peas during the last 5 minutes of cooking.
5. Add the cooked pasta to the eggplant mixture and toss over medium-high heat for 2 minutes. Serve hot, sprinkled with mozzarella or Parmesan.

NUTRITION PER SERVING

Calories 390 • Fat 12 g • Fiber 8 g • Protein 11 g • Carbohydrates 60 g

# pesto pasta with sun-dried tomatoes

MAKES 4 SERVINGS

When fresh tomatoes look pale and unappealing during the winter months, try this pasta. The sun-dried tomatoes and fresh basil will have you thinking that it's summer.

**8 ounces pasta (we recommend rotelle)**
**¼ cup extra-virgin olive oil**
**2 tablespoons water**
**2 cups fresh basil leaves**
**1 garlic clove, chopped**
**⅓ cup grated Parmesan cheese**
**½ cup thinly sliced sun-dried tomatoes**

1. Bring a large pot of water to a boil. Salt the water and add the pasta; cook according to the package directions. Drain and set aside.
2. While the pasta is cooking, combine the oil, water, basil, garlic, and ¼ cup of the Parmesan in a blender and purée.
3. Toss the puréed pesto with the pasta, tomatoes, and remaining Parmesan. Serve hot.

NUTRITION PER SERVING

Calories 380 • Fat 17 g • Fiber 3 g • Protein 12 g • Carbohydrates 47 g

# shrimp and pasta with feta

MAKES 4 SERVINGS

This recipe makes a great meal for guests and dates.

- 8 ounces spaghetti or linguine
- 2 teaspoons extra-virgin olive oil
- 3 garlic cloves, minced
- 1 cup chopped onion
- 2 cups tomato sauce
- 1 medium tomato, chopped
- Dried oregano
- Dried basil
- ½ cup white wine
- 1 pound raw shrimp, shelled and deveined
- ½ cup crumbled feta cheese

1. Bring a large pot of water to a boil. Salt the water and add the pasta; cook according to the package directions. Drain and set aside.
2. While the pasta is cooking, heat the oil in a large skillet over medium heat. Add the garlic and onion and sauté until the onion is translucent. Add the tomato sauce, chopped tomato, and a dash of oregano and basil, and cook until warmed through.
3. Add the white wine to the skillet and heat until the mixture is bubbling. Add the shrimp and cook until pink, 5 to 7 minutes.
4. Toss the sauce and shrimp with the hot pasta and top with feta.

NUTRITION PER SERVING

Calories 480 • Fat 10 g • Fiber 5 g • Protein 36 g • Carbohydrates 58 g

# roasted cauliflower, green olive, and almond pasta

MAKES 4 TO 6 SERVINGS

This may seem like an odd mix, but the combination of sweet caramelized cauliflower, nutty almonds, and delicately briny olives is fantastic! If you have leftovers, all the better, because this pasta tastes even better the next day.

**1 large head cauliflower, washed and chopped into small pieces**
**¼ cup extra-virgin olive oil, plus extra for roasting the cauliflower**
**Salt and freshly ground black pepper (sea salt is best)**
**1 cup (or more) fresh parsley leaves**
**½–¾ cup pitted green olives**
**½ cup toasted almonds (see Toasting Nuts on page 189)**
**1 pound pasta (capellini is a good choice)**
**Freshly grated Parmesan cheese**

1. Preheat the oven to 450°F.
2. Toss the cauliflower with a little olive oil until evenly coated. Spread the florets over a baking sheet and sprinkle with salt and pepper. Roast the cauliflower for 30 to 40 minutes, until the florets are golden brown and tender, flipping them with a spoon every 10 minutes or so to ensure even cooking.
3. While the cauliflower is roasting, combine the parsley, ¼ cup olive oil, olives, and almonds in a food processor, and blend until the ingredients are thoroughly combined and the olives and almonds are chopped well. Season with salt and pepper to taste.
4. Bring a large pot of water to a boil. Salt the water and add the pasta; cook according to the package directions until the pasta is al dente. Drain.
5. Toss the pasta with the roasted cauliflower and the parsley mixture. Season again with salt and pepper if necessary, then serve sprinkled with Parmesan.

NUTRITION PER SERVING

Calories 460 • Fat 17 g • Fiber 6 g • Protein 16 g • Carbohydrates 64 g

# orecchiette with broccoli rabe and pine nuts

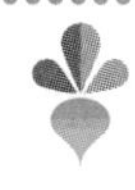

MAKES 4 TO 6 SERVINGS

A healthy, low-fat vegetarian recipe with a good amount of protein. Broccoli rabe is, as its name implies, a lot like broccoli, though darker in color, slightly more bitter in flavor, and with a leafier top. It's popular in Italian cooking.

**1 pound pasta (orecchiette works best)**
**1 pound broccoli rabe**
**1 tablespoon extra-virgin olive oil**
**2 garlic cloves, minced**
**¼ cup water**
**½ teaspoon salt (sea salt is best)**
**¼ teaspoon freshly ground black pepper**
**½ cup ricotta cheese**
**⅓ cup pine nuts**
**⅓ cup grated Parmesan cheese, plus extra for serving**

1. Bring a large pot of water to a boil. Salt the water and add the pasta; cook according to the package directions. Drain and set aside.
2. While the pasta is cooking, trim any tough lower stalks from the broccoli rabe. Wash the greens and chop them into bite-size pieces.
3. Heat the olive oil in a large skillet over medium heat. Add the garlic and sauté for 1 minute, until golden brown. Add the broccoli rabe and water to the skillet, reduce the heat to medium-low, cover, and steam the broccoli rabe for 2 to 4 minutes, until just tender, stirring occasionally. Season with salt and pepper.
4. Toss the pasta, broccoli rabe mixture, ricotta, pine nuts, and Parmesan together. Serve immediately, with extra Parmesan sprinkled on top.

NUTRITION PER SERVING

Calories 410 • Fat 10 g • Fiber 3 g • Protein 18 g • Carbohydrates 63 g

# baked ziti

MAKES 4 SERVINGS

A satisfying, baked version of the American chop suey you may have eaten as a child.

- **8 ounces ziti**
- **½ pound lean ground beef**
- **½ yellow onion, finely chopped**
- **2 garlic cloves, minced**
- **2 cups tomato sauce**
- **Dried oregano**
- **Dried basil**
- **Salt**
- **1 cup shredded mozzarella cheese**

1. Preheat the oven to 350°F.
2. Bring a large pot of water to a boil. Salt the water and add the ziti; cook according to the package directions. Drain and set aside.
3. While the ziti is cooking, heat a large skillet over medium heat. Add the beef, onion, and garlic and sauté until the beef is browned. Stir in the tomato sauce and oregano, basil, and salt to taste.
4. Mix the ziti with the sauce and cheese in a casserole dish, saving some cheese to sprinkle on top. Cover with aluminum foil and bake for 20 minutes, until the cheese is melted and bubbling.

NUTRITION PER SERVING

Calories 390 • Fat 8 g • Fiber 3 g • Protein 28 g • Carbohydrates 50 g

# lazy pasta

MAKES 4 SERVINGS

Sauté the vegetables while the pasta cooks for a quick, vegetable-rich meal in minutes.

**8 ounces pasta**
**3 teaspoons butter**
**1 small zucchini, sliced**
**6 mushrooms, wiped clean and quartered**
**1 tomato, diced**
**¼ cup grated Parmesan cheese**
**1½ teaspoons skim milk**

1. Bring a large pot of water to a boil. Salt the water and add the pasta; cook according to the package directions. Drain and set aside.
2. While the pasta is cooking, melt 2 teaspoons of the butter in a large skillet over medium heat. Add the zucchini and mushrooms and sauté until soft, about 7 minutes. Add the tomato and cook for 1 minute longer.
3. Melt the remaining teaspoon of butter in the hot pasta. Add the Parmesan, milk, and vegetables. Toss well and serve.

NUTRITION PER SERVING

Calories 310 • Fat 6 g • Fiber 3 g • Protein 14 g • Carbohydrates 51 g

# matt's potcheese and noodles

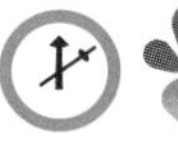
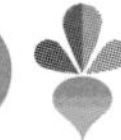

MAKES 4 SERVINGS

Quick, creamy, cheap, and tasty, these noodles qualify as serious comfort food.

**8 ounces egg noodles**
**2 tablespoons butter**
**1 large onion, sliced**
**½ of a (16-ounce) container fat-free cottage cheese**
**Salt and freshly ground black pepper**

1. Bring a large pot of water to a boil. Salt the water and add noodles; cook according to the package directions. Drain and set aside.
2. While the noodles are cooking, melt the butter in a skillet over medium heat. Add the onion and sauté until translucent. Mix in the cottage cheese and heat gently until warmed through.
3. Combine the cottage-cheese sauce and noodles in a serving bowl and mix well. Season with salt and pepper to taste and serve hot.

NUTRITION PER SERVING
Calories 310 • Fat 7 g • Fiber 2 g • Protein 13 g • Carbohydrates 49 g

# orzo with diced ham and vegetables

MAKES 4 SERVINGS

This quick pasta dish is delicious hot or cold.

- **1¼ cups orzo**
- **1 teaspoon extra-virgin olive oil**
- **⅓ cup finely chopped onion**
- **1 cup diced cooked ham**
- **⅓ cup corn kernels (fresh or frozen)**
- **⅓ cup green beans, chopped into ½-inch lengths**
- **3 tablespoons Dijon mustard**
- **2 tablespoons nonfat plain yogurt**
- **2 tablespoons red wine vinegar**

1. Bring a large pot of water to a boil. Salt the water and add the orzo; cook according to the package directions. Drain and set aside.
2. While the orzo is cooking, heat the oil in a large skillet over medium heat. Add the onion and sauté until softened, about 5 minutes. Add the ham and cook for 3 minutes longer. Add the corn and green beans; cook for 4 minutes longer.
3. Add the orzo to the ham and vegetables mixture. Stir in the mustard, yogurt, and vinegar; mix thoroughly. Serve hot.

NUTRITION PER SERVING

Calories 390 • Fat 10 g • Fiber 4 g • Protein 21 g • Carbohydrates 52 g

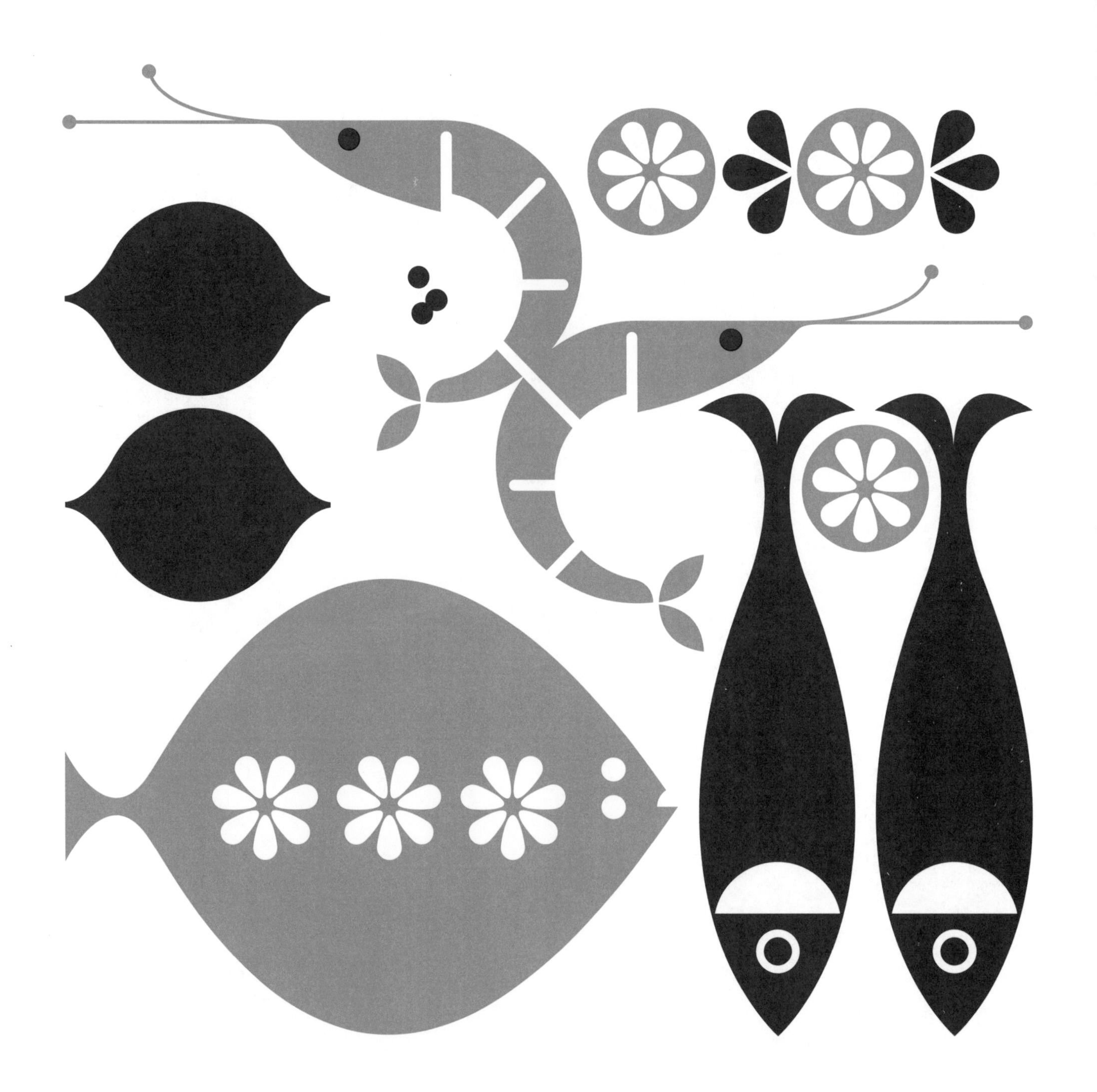

# chapter 7

## the best of seafood

Although it's true that some people just plain don't like fish, we find the idea incredibly hard to believe. The usual complaint is "Fish is just too fishy." Not true! While some varieties have a stronger fish flavor than others, fish is, for the most part, light and healthy with a mild flavor. We suggest you give it a chance. Compared to beef, pork, and chicken (and especially when you take into account hefty bones and the extra fat that has to be trimmed off for those cuts of meat), many kinds of fish are relatively inexpensive as well as quick to prepare and easy to clean up. To make life a lot simpler, we have included a number of great oven and microwave tips for poaching fish.

When buying fish, always make sure that it's very fresh. Don't buy fish that is discolored in any way. Check the expiration date and smell the fish before cooking it (good advice for any type of meat).

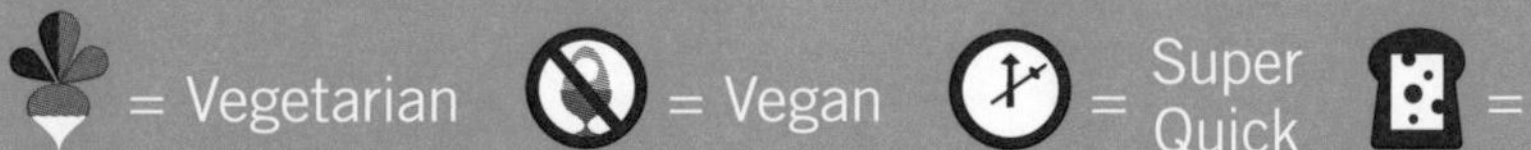
= Vegetarian  = Vegan  = Super Quick = Dorm Room Favorite

# brett's versatile fish steak

MAKES 4 SERVINGS

If you have a barbecue grill and are in the mood, you can grill this fish steak over fire. A George Foreman Grill will also do the trick.

**1½ pounds fish, cut as steaks (we recommend tuna or swordfish)**
**1 cup vinaigrette of choice**

1. Marinate the fish in the vinaigrette for 2 hours in the refrigerator.
2. Preheat your grill.
3. Grill the fish for about 5 minutes per side, checking often, until the steak is done to your satisfaction. If you like your tuna rare, grilling time will be only 2 to 3 minutes per side.

NUTRITION PER SERVING

Calories 420 • Fat 28 g • Fiber 0 g • Protein 32 g • Carbohydrates 8 g

# light lime-garlic shrimp

MAKES 4 SERVINGS

A spicy shrimp preparation that's delicious with hot rice and a green vegetable.

**2 tablespoons lime juice**
**2 garlic cloves, thickly sliced**
**1 tablespoon hot sauce**
**½ teaspoon salt**
**1½–2 pounds shrimp, peeled and deveined**

1. Preheat the oven to 350°F.
2. Combine the lime juice, garlic, hot sauce, and salt in a small bowl; mix well.
3. Line a casserole dish with aluminum foil so that there is enough extra at each end to fold back over the dish. Place the shrimp in the dish, pour the lime mixture over the shrimp, fold in the ends of the foil to cover the shrimp, and bake for 7 minutes.

NUTRITION PER SERVING

Calories 180 • Fat 3 g • Fiber 0 g • Protein 35 g • Carbohydrates 3 g

# lime-basil mahi mahi steaks

MAKES 2 SERVINGS

This marinade also works well with halibut or swordfish.

**¼ cup lime juice**
**1½ tablespoons chopped fresh basil**
**1 teaspoon freshly ground black pepper**
**1 teaspoon minced garlic**
**½ teaspoon salt**
**2 mahi mahi steaks**

1. Combine the lime juice, basil, pepper, garlic, and salt in a ziplock bag. Add the mahi mahi steaks and seal, squeezing out as much air as possible. Marinate the steaks in the refrigerator for 30 to 60 minutes.
2. Preheat your oven or toaster oven to 375°F.
3. Remove the fish from the ziplock bag and place it, together with some of the marinade, on a small tray with raised edges. Bake for 12 to 15 minutes, or until the fish begins to flake.

NUTRITION PER SERVING

Calories 190 • Fat 1.5 g • Fiber 0 g • Protein 38 g • Carbohydrates 4 g

# festive flounder

MAKES 4 SERVINGS

Even your friends who claim not to like fish will like this dish.

- ¼ cup all-purpose flour
- ½ teaspoon freshly ground black pepper
- 4 (6-ounce) flounder fillets
- 1 tablespoon extra-virgin olive oil
- 1 tablespoon butter
- 10 mushrooms, wiped clean and sliced
- 3 scallions, sliced
- 2 garlic cloves, minced
- 1 lemon, cut in half

1. Combine the flour and pepper on a large plate.
2. Pat the fish fillets dry with paper towels. One fillet at a time, coat each thoroughly with the flour mixture.
3. Heat the oil in a large skillet over medium-high heat. Cook the fillets (2 at a time, if possible) for 2 minutes per side, flipping only once.
4. Melt the butter in another large skillet over medium heat. Add the mushrooms, scallions, and garlic. Turn the heat to medium-high after 2 minutes and sauté, stirring often, for 7 to 8 minutes. Add the juice of 1 lemon half to the pan and remove from heat.
5. Pour the vegetable mixture evenly over the fillets. Slice the remaining lemon half into 4 wedges and serve with the fish.

NUTRITION PER SERVING

Calories 260 • Fat 9 g • Fiber 1 g • Protein 34 g • Carbohydrates 10 g

# tuna with tomato, onion, and parsley salsa

MAKES 4 SERVINGS

This salsa is also delicious spooned over a simple chicken breast.

**4 large tomatoes, peeled, seeded, and finely chopped**
**1 small red onion, finely chopped**
**1 garlic clove, minced**
**2 tablespoons chopped fresh parsley**
**½ teaspoon salt**
**1 tablespoon red wine vinegar**
**4 tuna steaks**

1. Combine the tomatoes, onion, garlic, parsley, salt, and vinegar in a small bowl and mix well. Chill.
2. Preheat the broiler. Place the tuna on a baking sheet or broiler pan. Broil to desired doneness, 5 to 8 minutes per side. Serve with a scoop of the chilled salsa.

NUTRITION PER SERVING

Calories 290 • Fat 9 g • Fiber 3 g • Protein 42 g • Carbohydrates 10 g

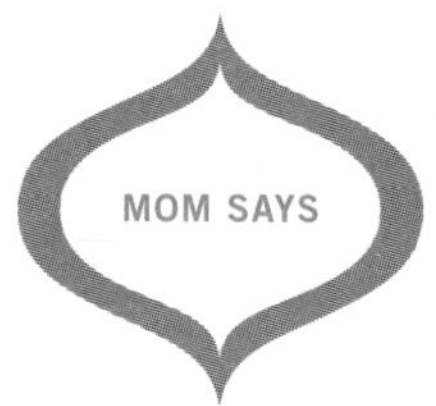


## quick cleanup

When broiling fish, placing it on aluminum foil instead of directly on the broiler rack minimizes cleanup.

# sole with orange sauce

MAKES 4 SERVINGS

Reduced orange juice makes a delicious sauce for all kinds of white fish. Add a dash of cayenne or Tabasco if you like.

**½ tablespoon butter**
**½ tablespoon all-purpose flour**
**½ teaspoon grated orange zest**
**¾ cup orange juice**
**1½ pounds sole fillets**
**1 lemon, cut into 6 wedges**

1. Melt the butter in a saucepan over medium heat. Whisk in the flour and cook for 1 minute. Add the orange zest and juice and cook, stirring often, until the sauce begins to thicken. Turn the heat to high and cook, stirring, for 1 to 2 minutes longer to thicken the sauce.
2. Place the fillets in a microwave-safe dish (you may need to do this in several batches) and squeeze the juice from 2 lemon wedges over them.
3. Cover the dish and microwave on high for 2 to 3 minutes. After the first minute, check the fish every 30 seconds, as the amount of cooking time will depend on the thickness of the fillets and how many you put in the microwave at a time. When the centers of the fillets are opaque, they're done.
4. Pour the orange sauce over the fillets and serve with lemon wedges.

NUTRITION PER SERVING

Calories 240 • Fat 4.5 g • Fiber 0 g • Protein 39 g • Carbohydrates 7 g

# red snapper and capers

MAKES 4 SERVINGS

Capers add a juicy saltiness to this dish, without the added fat of olives.

- **2 teaspoons grated lemon zest**
- **3 tablespoons lemon juice**
- **⅓ cup small capers**
- **1 tablespoon water**
- **4 garlic cloves, minced**
- **Pinch of salt**
- **Pinch of freshly ground black pepper**
- **1½ pounds red snapper fillets**

1. Preheat the oven to 425°F.
2. Combine the lemon zest and juice, capers, water, garlic, salt, and pepper in a mixing bowl. Stir well.
3. Place the snapper fillets in a glass baking dish and pour the juice mixture over them. Bake for 7 to 10 minutes (the cooking time will depend on the thickness of fillets), until the fillets are flaky and of a uniform texture throughout.

NUTRITION PER SERVING

Calories 180 • Fat 2.5 g • Fiber 1 g • Protein 35 g • Carbohydrates 2 g

## what's a caper?

Capers are the buds of a flower found in the Mediterranean and Asia. They are sun-dried and then pickled.

# breaded whitefish

MAKES 4 SERVINGS

A fresh take on frozen fish sticks. Server with tartar sauce if you like.

**¼ cup all-purpose flour**
**1 egg**
**1 tablespoon water**
**1 cup breadcrumbs**
**1 teaspoon dried sage**
**1 teaspoon dried thyme**
**1 teaspoon freshly ground black pepper**
**½ teaspoon salt**
**½ teaspoon cayenne pepper**
**1½ pounds whitefish, such as cod, haddock, or flounder**

1. Preheat the oven to 350°F. Place a flat wire rack on a baking sheet.
2. Spread the flour on a plate. Beat together the egg and water in a small dish. Combine the breadcrumbs and seasonings in another small dish.
3. Rinse the fish and pat dry. Dip the fish into the flour, turning to coat, then dip the fish into the egg mixture, thoroughly coating it. Finally, dip the fish into the breadcrumb mixture, patting the mixture onto the fish to completely cover it.
4. Place the breaded fish on the rack in the baking pan. Bake for about 25 minutes (the exact time will vary depending on the thickness of the fish), until it's cooked through.

NUTRITION PER SERVING

Calories 310 • Fat 4 g • Fiber 2 g • Protein 38 g • Carbohydrates 27 g

# quick cod

MAKES 4 SERVINGS

Your microwave is perfect for cooking fresh mild fish, keeping it moist without added fat.

**1½ pounds cod, cut into 4 portions**
**2 lemons**
**Freshly ground black pepper**

1. Arrange the cod in a microwave-safe glass dish. Sprinkle with the juice from 1 lemon and pepper to taste.
2. Cover and microwave on high for 2 to 3 minutes. Check the doneness of the fish after 2 minutes. If the fish is almost done, cover it and let it sit for a minute to finish cooking, rather than microwaving for another minute. Serve with the remaining lemon, cut into wedges.

NUTRITION PER SERVING
Calories 140 • Fat 1 g • Fiber 0 g • Protein 30 g • Carbohydrates 0 g

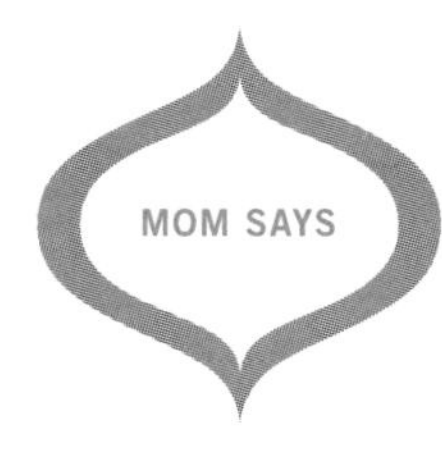


## don't let it hang around!

Fresh or defrosted fish should be kept in the coldest area of your refrigerator. Cook within 2 days. You can stock up on an extra serving or two of fish when it's on sale. Wrap it well in plastic wrap, place in a ziplock freezer bag and freeze for no more than one month.

# garlic-ginger scallops

MAKES 4 SERVINGS

Serve these slightly spicy scallops over a bed of hot rice.

**½ teaspoon extra-virgin olive oil**
**2 garlic cloves, minced**
**1 teaspoon freshly grated ginger**
**Pinch of crushed red pepper flakes or cayenne pepper**
**1½ pounds small scallops**
**¼ cup water**
**3 tablespoons chopped fresh parsley**
**Salt and freshly ground black pepper**

1. Heat the oil in a large skillet over medium heat. Add the garlic, ginger, and red pepper flakes and sauté for 20 seconds. Add the scallops and water and simmer until the scallops are opaque, about 5 minutes.

2. Remove from the heat and stir in the parsley and salt and pepper to taste.

NUTRITION PER SERVING

Calories 290 • Fat 2.5 g • Fiber 0 g • Protein 55 g • Carbohydrates 11 g

# honey dijon salmon

MAKES 4 SERVINGS

Mustard and salmon always make a good pair.

**2 tablespoons Dijon mustard**
**4 teaspoons honey**
**2 teaspoons chopped fresh parsley**
**¼ cup breadcrumbs**
**4 (4-ounce) salmon fillets**
**4 lemon wedges**

1. Preheat the oven to 450°F.
2. Mix together the mustard and honey in a small bowl.
3. In a separate bowl, combine the parsley and breadcrumbs.
4. Place the salmon in a baking dish. Spread the mustard mixture evenly over each fillet and sprinkle the breadcrumb mixture on top. Bake for 10 minutes for each inch of thickness, or until the fish is flaky. Serve with lemon wedges.

NUTRITION PER SERVING

Calories 260 • Fat 8 g • Fiber 1 g • Protein 24 g • Carbohydrates 13 g

# slow-cooker citrus salmon

MAKES 2 SERVINGS

This dish looks fancy but it's very easy to prepare.

**2 (4-ounce) salmon fillets**
**1 cup orange juice**
**2 tablespoons lime juice**
**2 tablespoons lemon juice**
**1 teaspoon minced fresh thyme or ¼ teaspoon dried thyme**
**¼ teaspoon salt**
**¼ teaspoon freshly ground black pepper**
**Hot cooked brown rice**

1. Place the salmon fillets in a slow cooker. Combine the orange, lime, and lemon juices, and pour over the salmon. Season with thyme, salt, and pepper.
2. Cover and cook on the high setting for 20 to 30 minutes, or until the salmon is opaque and flakes easily. Serve with brown rice.

NUTRITION PER SERVING
Calories 250 • Fat 8 g • Fiber 0 g • Protein 27 g • Carbohydrates 16 g

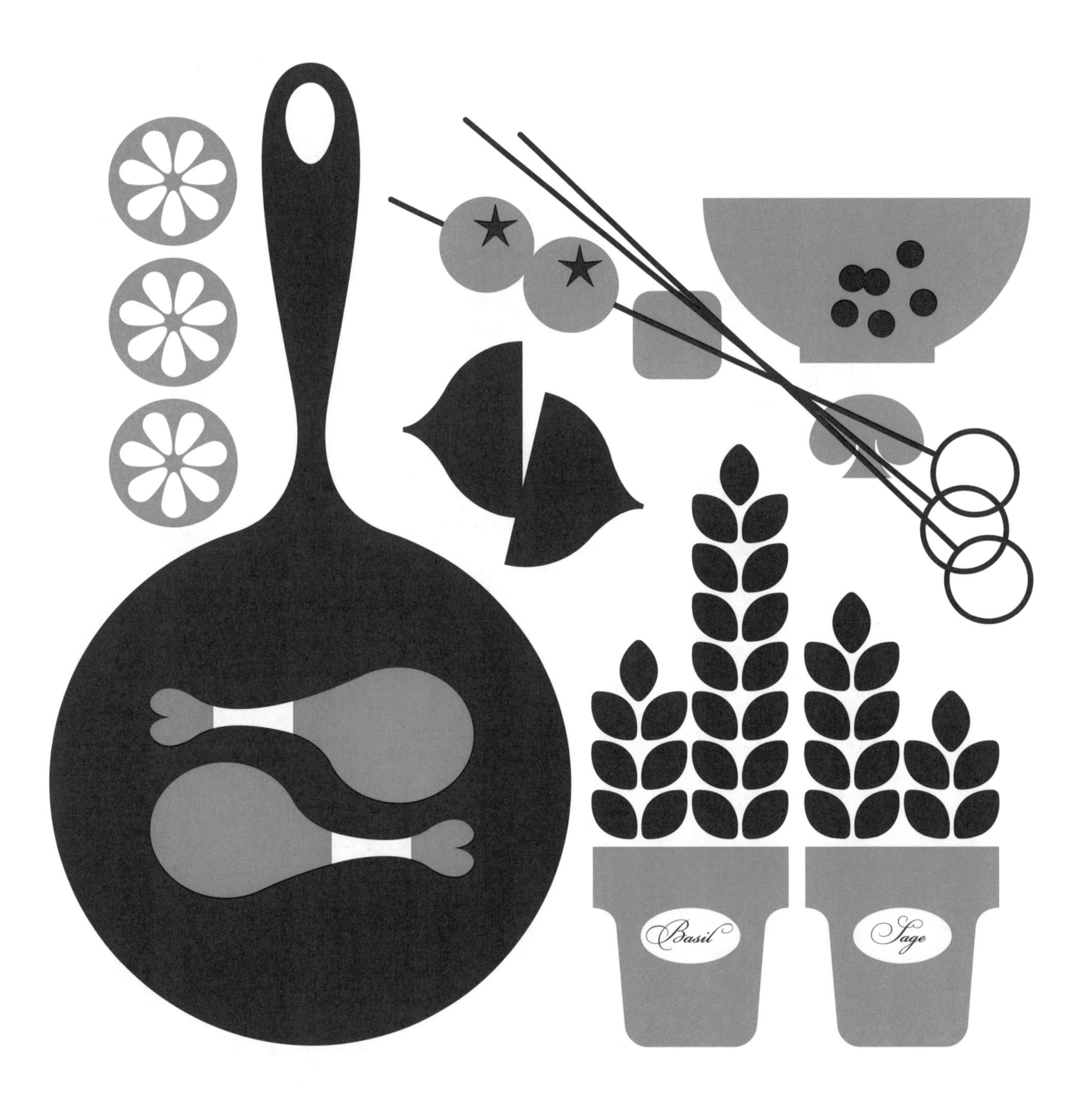
Basil
Sage

# chapter 8

## simple chicken dinners

Chicken is easy to prepare, it's perfect for lunch or dinner, and its leftovers can be used in a variety of dishes. Most of our recipes call for boneless, skinless chicken breasts, but thighs and legs can often be substituted, and they cost less, as well. Preparation usually involves no more than chopping up a few ingredients, throwing them in a pan with the chicken, and adding an easy sauce. The most time-consuming part of the process is the actual cooking time. Please note: What most of us consider to be a chicken breast is actually a half-breast; chicken breasts are made up of two pieces. Just to be clear, we've called for half-breasts in our recipes.

As with all raw meat, chicken can carry dangerous bacteria. You'll be fine as long as you are conscientious about rinsing raw chicken in cold water before cooking it (pat it dry afterward) and cleaning your utensils, preparation area, and hands with hot suds after handling raw chicken.

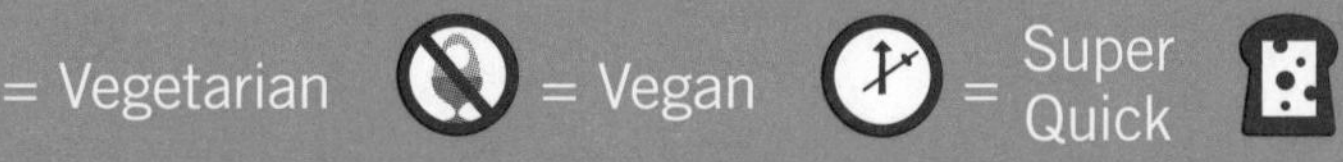

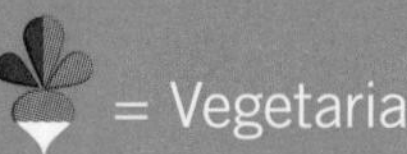
= Vegetarian

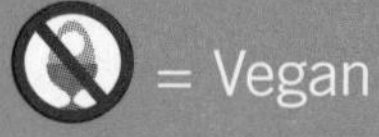
= Vegan

= Super Quick

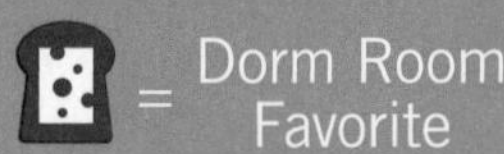
= Dorm Room Favorite

# sweet orange chicken

MAKES 4 SERVINGS

This one gets five stars. Great hot or cold — though it's usually all gone before it has a chance to cool off.

**4 boneless, skinless chicken breast halves**
**4 teaspoons Dijon mustard**
**½ medium onion, diced**
**1 cup orange juice**
**2 teaspoons butter**
**2 tablespoons packed brown sugar**

1. Preheat the oven to 350°F.
2. Place the chicken in a baking dish and spread mustard evenly over each piece. Sprinkle the onion over the chicken, pour orange juice over all, and place ½-teaspoon morsels of butter near each piece of chicken. Bake uncovered for 25 minutes.
3. Flip the chicken and sprinkle sugar evenly over each piece. Bake for 10 minutes longer, or until cooked through (no pink shows in the middle).

NUTRITION PER SERVING
Calories 210 • Fat 3.5 g • Fiber 0 g • Protein 28 g • Carbohydrates 14 g

# honey mustard and garlic chicken

MAKES 4 SERVINGS

If you have leftovers, slice the chicken and add it to a big green salad.

**¼ cup honey**
**½ cup Dijon mustard**
**4 boneless, skinless chicken breast halves**
**1 garlic clove, cut into slivers**

1. Preheat the oven to 350°F.
2. Mix together the honey and mustard.
3. Make 4 small cuts in the center of each piece of chicken, then arrange the chicken in a baking dish. Insert a sliver of garlic into each cut. Spread the honey-mustard mixture over each breast.
4. Bake for 30 minutes, basting the chicken once or twice with any accumulated pan sauce. Transfer the chicken to a preheated broiler (or turn the oven temperature up to broil) and broil for 5 minutes, until the tops are crisp (but not burnt).

NUTRITION PER SERVING

Calories 220 • Fat 1.5 g • Fiber 0 g • Protein 27 g • Carbohydrates 23 g

# apple chicken

MAKES 4 SERVINGS

Apple and mushrooms may seem like an odd combination, but give it a try. College is all about new experiences.

**1 tablespoon extra-virgin olive oil**
**4 boneless, skinless chicken breast halves**
**1 cup applesauce (see page 235 for our recipe)**
**Salt**
**8 medium mushrooms, wiped clean and sliced**
**Freshly ground black pepper**

1. Preheat the oven to 350°F.
2. Heat the oil in a large skillet over medium heat. Add the chicken and cook until browned lightly on both sides.
3. Place the browned chicken in a casserole dish and cover evenly with applesauce. Sprinkle with ¼ teaspoon salt, cover, and bake for 25 minutes.
4. Add the mushrooms to the casserole dish. Cover and bake for 10 minutes longer. Season with salt and pepper.

NUTRITION PER SERVING
Calories 200 • Fat 5 g • Fiber 1 g • Protein 28 g • Carbohydrates 8 g

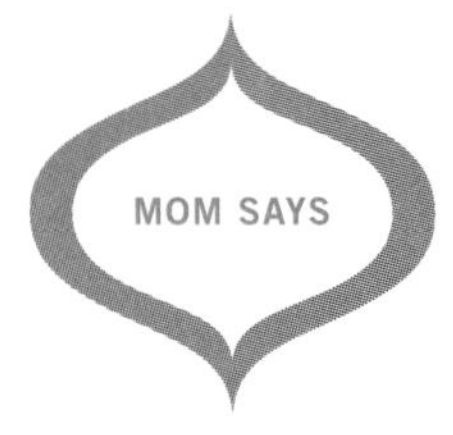


## making do

If your casserole dish doesn't have a cover, use aluminum foil to cover it instead.

## chicken with green peppers

MAKES 4 SERVINGS

While this is good hot, it's even better cold. Make lots to keep in the refrigerator as leftovers.

**4 boneless, skinless chicken breast halves**
**2 green bell peppers, seeded and chopped**
**⅓ cup low-sodium soy sauce**

1. Preheat the oven to 350°F.
2. Arrange the chicken and peppers in a large baking dish. Pour soy sauce over everything.
3. Cover and bake for 30 minutes, or until chicken is cooked through.

NUTRITION PER SERVING
Calories 150 • Fat 1.5 g • Fiber 1 g • Protein 29 g • Carbohydrates 3 g

## apricot chicken

MAKES 4 SERVINGS

**2 tablespoons apricot jam**
**⅓ cup low-sodium soy sauce**
**1 tablespoon freshly grated ginger**
**4 boneless, skinless chicken breast halves**

1. Mix the jam, soy sauce, and ginger in a baking dish or ziplock bag. Add the chicken and marinate in the refrigerator for at least 3 hours.
2. Preheat the oven to 350°F. Bake the chicken for 30 minutes, or until cooked through (no pink shows in the middle).

NUTRITION PER SERVING
Calories 170 • Fat 1.5 g • Fiber 0 g • Protein 29 g • Carbohydrates 9 g

# chicken pesto pasta

MAKES 5 SERVINGS

Williams College, located in western Massachusetts, and Amherst College, in central Massachusetts, have long been rivals — Amherst was founded long ago by a split-off faction of professors and students from Williams. Nevertheless, even as Williams students we must commend our rivals for contributing an exceptional recipe. Maybe they got it from one of our library books.

**2 cups lightly packed fresh basil leaves**
**⅓ cup grated Parmesan cheese**
**3 garlic cloves, minced**
**½ teaspoon salt**
**½ teaspoon freshly ground black pepper**
**½ cup plus 1 teaspoon extra-virgin olive oil**
**8 ounces penne**
**3 boneless, skinless chicken breast halves, cut into strips**

1. In a food processor or blender, combine the basil, Parmesan, garlic, salt, and pepper; finely chop. Add ½ cup of the olive oil and blend until smooth.
2. Bring a large pot of water to a boil. Salt the water and add the pasta; cook according to the package directions. Drain.
3. Heat the remaining teaspoon of oil in a skillet over medium heat. Add the chicken and sauté about 10 minutes, or until cooked through (no pink shows in the middle).
4. Pour the pesto sauce over the drained pasta, add the chicken, and mix well. Serve warm or cold.

NUTRITION PER SERVING

Calories 530 • Fat 31 g • Fiber 1 g • Protein 24 g • Carbohydrates 34 g

# italian chicken sauté

MAKES 2 SERVINGS

For faster cooking, you can slice the raw chicken and sauté the strips. Serve over rice.

**2 tablespoons freshly minced garlic**
**½ cup Italian dressing (or ¼ cup olive oil plus ¼ cup lemon juice)**
**2 boneless, skinless chicken breast halves**
**½ teaspoon salt**
**½ teaspoon freshly ground black pepper**

1. Combine the garlic and Italian dressing in a ziplock bag. Place the chicken breasts in the bag, seal, and marinate in the refrigerator for at least 30 minutes and up to several hours.
2. Warm a skillet over medium heat. Add the chicken breasts and marinade, and season with salt and pepper. Cook for 5 to 8 minutes on each side, until golden brown and no longer pink inside.

**NOTE:** You can also use a George Foreman Grill to prepare this recipe: Grill the marinated chicken breasts (discard the marinade) seasoned with salt and pepper. The total cooking time will range from 8 to 12 minutes, depending on how thick the chicken breasts are.

NUTRITION PER SERVING
Calories 200 • Fat 3.5 g • Fiber 0 g • Protein 28 g • Carbohydrates 8 g

# chicken with artichokes

MAKES 4 SERVINGS

This is a tasty and substantial recipe for all you artichoke lovers out there. It's best served over rice or pasta.

- **1 tablespoon extra-virgin olive oil**
- **1 small yellow onion, chopped**
- **1 green bell pepper, seeded and chopped**
- **2 teaspoons dried basil**
- **2 teaspoons minced garlic**
- **1 (14.5-ounce) can chopped, stewed tomatoes, drained**
- **2 boneless, skinless chicken breast halves, cut into bite-size chunks**
- **½ teaspoon salt**
- **1 teaspoon freshly ground black pepper**
- **1 (14-ounce) can artichoke hearts in water, drained**

1. Heat the oil in a large skillet over medium heat. Add the onion and green pepper and sauté for 5 minutes.
2. Stir in the basil, garlic, tomatoes, chicken, salt, and pepper. Reduce the heat and simmer until the chicken is cooked through (no pink shows in the middle), about 15 minutes.
3. Add the artichoke hearts and continue simmering until heated through.

NUTRITION PER SERVING

Calories 200 • Fat 4.5 g • Fiber 5 g • Protein 19 g • Carbohydrates 21 g

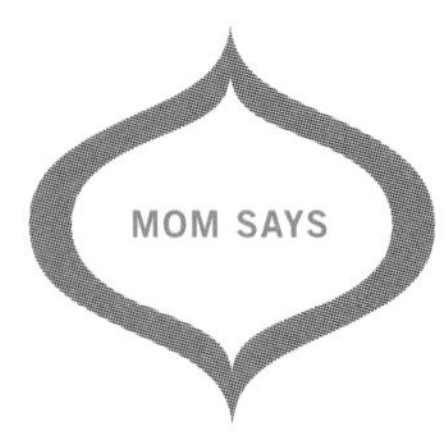


## quick test

When frying or sautéing in oil, to test whether the oil is hot enough, flick a drop of water into the skillet. If it spatters, the oil is ready. If not, keep heating.

# lemon-pepper chicken and artichokes

MAKES 6 SERVINGS

This dish is simple, light, and good-looking — a sure bet for impressing your friends with your culinary ability.

- **1 tablespoon extra-virgin olive oil**
- **1 tablespoon chopped garlic**
- **1 teaspoon crushed red pepper flakes**
- **4 boneless, skinless chicken breast halves, cut into 1-inch pieces**
- **1 teaspoon dried thyme**
- **2 (14-ounce) cans artichoke hearts in water, drained**
- **¼ cup white wine**
- **1 (2.25-ounce) can sliced black olives, drained**
- **1 tablespoon capers**
- **3 tablespoons lemon juice**
- **½ teaspoon lemon-pepper seasoning**
- **¼ cup crumbled goat cheese (optional)**
- **30 grape tomatoes, halved**
- **4 leaves fresh basil, chopped**
- **4 leaves fresh mint, chopped**
- **6 lemon wedges for serving**

1. Heat the oil in a large skillet over medium-high heat. Add the garlic and red pepper flakes and sauté for 1 minute. Add the chicken pieces and season with thyme. Toss the chicken to coat and sauté for 6 to 7 minutes, until no longer pink on the outside.
2. Add the artichokes and wine to the skillet. Stir gently and cook for 5 minutes longer, allowing the wine to reduce and the chicken to cook thoroughly.
3. Turn off the heat. Add the olives, capers, lemon juice, lemon-pepper seasoning, and goat cheese, if using. Toss gently. Top the dish with grape tomatoes and chopped basil and mint. Garnish each serving with a lemon wedge. Buon appetito!

NUTRITION PER SERVING

Calories 230 • Fat 5 g • Fiber 7 g • Protein 24 g • Carbohydrates 21 g

# lemon chicken

MAKES 4 SERVINGS

A classic combination — simple and delicious.

**4 garlic cloves, minced**
**2 lemons**
**Salt**
**½ teaspoon freshly ground black pepper**
**4 boneless, skinless chicken breast halves**

1. Preheat the oven to 350°F.
2. Combine the garlic, juice from 1½ of the lemons, salt to taste, and pepper in a casserole dish. Add the chicken breasts and spoon some of the juice over each. Cut the remaining lemon half into 4 slices and place 1 slice on top of each chicken breast.
3. Bake for 30 minutes, or until the chicken is cooked through (no pink shows in the middle).

NUTRITION PER SERVING

Calories 140 • Fat 1.5 g • Fiber 1 g • Protein 27 g • Carbohydrates 3 g

# sesame chicken

MAKES 4 SERVINGS

This chicken is also delicious as the star of a main-course salad.

**4 boneless, skinless chicken breast halves**
**4 tablespoons honey**
**3 tablespoons sesame seeds**
**1 teaspoon garlic powder**
**½ teaspoon freshly ground black pepper**

1. Preheat the oven to 350°F.
2. Arrange the chicken in a single layer in a casserole dish. Warm the honey slightly in a microwave or small saucepan over low heat and then brush it evenly over the chicken.
3. Combine the sesame seeds, garlic powder, and pepper in a small bowl, and sprinkle the mixture evenly over the chicken. Bake uncovered for 30 minutes, or until the chicken is cooked through (no pink shows in the middle).

NUTRITION PER SERVING

Calories 230 • Fat 4.5 g • Fiber 1 g • Protein 29 g • Carbohydrates 19 g

# homemade chinese takeout

MAKES 4 SERVINGS

If you're craving Chinese but want food that's better for you and less expensive, this is the recipe for you.

- **1 teaspoon sesame oil**
- **1 tablespoon olive oil**
- **2 garlic cloves, chopped**
- **1 teaspoon crushed red pepper flakes (or to taste)**
- **2 boneless, skinless chicken breast halves, cut into bite-size pieces (fine to use 8 ounces of thigh meat for additional flavor)**
- **1 bag frozen Asian-style mixed vegetables**
- **⅓ cup hoisin sauce**
- **¼ cup honey**
- **Ginger, freshly grated or ground**
- **Onion powder**
- **Garlic powder**
- **Salt and freshly ground black pepper**
- **Hot cooked brown rice**

1. Heat the oils in a large skillet or stockpot over medium heat. Add the garlic and red pepper flakes and sauté for 1 minute, until the garlic begins to brown.
2. Add the chicken and sauté 6 to 8 minutes, stirring often, until no longer pink on the inside.
3. Add the vegetables, hoisin, honey, and spices to taste. Continue to cook until the vegetables are tender.
4. Serve hot over cooked rice.

NUTRITION PER SERVING

Calories 250 • Fat 4 g • Fiber 2 g • Protein 17 g • Carbohydrates 39 g

## asian chicken salad wrap

MAKES 3 SERVINGS

Savory, crunchy, and portable.

- ¼ cup orange juice
- 3 tablespoons duck sauce
- 2 tablespoons sesame oil
- 3 cups shredded lettuce
- ¼ teaspoon ground ginger
- ¼ teaspoon salt
- ¼ teaspoon freshly ground black pepper
- 3 tablespoons roughly chopped peanuts
- 3 tablespoons Chinese-style crispy noodles (the noodles you often get with Chinese takeout work fine)
- 3 whole-grain sandwich wraps
- 1 boneless, skinless chicken breast half, cooked and cut into strips

1. Stir together the orange juice, duck sauce, and sesame oil in a small bowl.
2. Toss the shredded lettuce with the ginger, salt, and pepper. Dress with the orange juice mixture; add the nuts and crispy noodles and toss again.
3. Lay out the 3 wraps on plates. Divide the chicken strips among the wraps. Top with the dressed salad and roll up.

NUTRITION PER SERVING

Calories 240 • Fat 14 g • Fiber 2 g • Protein 13 g • Carbohydrates 17 g

### toasting nuts

To toast nuts or seeds, place them in a dry skillet over medium heat. Keep them moving in the pan, either by shaking it gently or turning them with a spatula, until they turn a golden brown. And keep a close eye on them — once they start to brown, they go from deliciously toasted to burnt very quickly.

# chicken santa fe

MAKES 2 SERVINGS

Make this dish as mild or as hot as you like. The quantity of hot sauce is up to you.

**2 teaspoons extra-virgin olive oil**
**2 boneless, skinless chicken breast halves**
**1 (15-ounce) can black beans, rinsed and drained**
**1 medium tomato, chopped**
**½ green bell pepper, seeded and chopped**
**Hot sauce**
**Ground cumin**
**1 teaspoon chopped fresh cilantro (optional)**

1. Heat the oil in a large skillet over medium heat. Add the chicken breasts and sauté until cooked through (no pink shows in the middle), 10 to 15 minutes.
2. In a saucepan over medium heat, warm the beans, tomato, and green pepper. Season to taste with hot sauce and cumin.
3. Place each chicken breast on a plate and smother with beans. Garnish with fresh cilantro, if using, and serve immediately.

NUTRITION PER SERVING

Calories 310 • Fat 6 g • Fiber 11 g • Protein 37 g • Carbohydrates 33 g

# slow-cooked chicken fiesta

MAKES 4 SERVINGS

This is a classic slow-cooker recipe that is easily adaptable to whatever you have on hand. Try adding green chiles, onions, garlic, or red and green bell peppers; substitute diced tomatoes and Mexican-style herbs for the salsa; and use kidney or pinto beans instead of black beans — it really doesn't matter!

**1 (12-ounce) jar salsa**
**4 boneless, skinless chicken breast halves, cut into 1-inch pieces**
**1 (15-ounce) can black beans, rinsed and drained**
**1 (16-ounce) can whole-kernel corn, drained, or 1 (16-ounce) package frozen corn**
**½ cup shredded cheddar or Monterey Jack cheese**
**¼ cup low-fat sour cream**

1. Drain some of the liquid from the salsa. Combine the salsa, chicken, and black beans in a slow cooker. Cover and cook on the low setting for 8 hours or on the high setting for 4 hours.
2. Add the corn 1 hour before the chicken is done.
3. Top with cheese and sour cream before serving. (The mixture is excellent wrapped in a tortilla!)

NUTRITION PER SERVING

Calories 330 • Fat 5 g • Fiber 8 g • Protein 38 g • Carbohydrates 32 g

# kelly's chicken and mushrooms

MAKES 4 SERVINGS

This chicken dish goes great with a plate of hot cooked rice.

- **½ cup all-purpose flour**
- **4 boneless, skinless chicken breast halves**
- **2 teaspoons extra-virgin olive oil**
- **1 onion, finely chopped**
- **2 garlic cloves, minced**
- **15 mushrooms, wiped clean and sliced**
- **1 cup white wine**
- **Salt and freshly ground black pepper**

1. Spread the flour on a plate. Dip the chicken breasts into the flour, thoroughly coating them. Set the chicken aside.
2. Heat the oil in a skillet over medium heat. Add the onion and garlic and sauté until the onion is translucent. Add the mushrooms and chicken to the pan and sauté until the chicken is cooked through (no pink shows in the middle), 10 to 15 minutes.
3. Add the wine to the skillet. Continue stirring until the sauce in the pan thickens, repeatedly spooning it over chicken breasts. Season with salt and pepper. Serve each chicken breast with a little sauce drizzled over it.

NUTRITION PER SERVING

Calories 290 • Fat 4 g • Fiber 2 g • Protein 32 g • Carbohydrates 19 g

# chicken and broccoli sauté

MAKES 4 SERVINGS

Serve this dish over a plate of rice for a complete meal.

**1 teaspoon extra-virgin olive oil**
**3 cups chopped broccoli**
**2 carrots, peeled and chopped**
**2 tablespoons finely chopped yellow onion**
**2 garlic cloves, minced**
**4 boneless, skinless chicken breast halves, cut into bite-size pieces**
**2 tablespoons teriyaki sauce (see page 249 for our recipe)**

1. Heat the oil in a large skillet over medium heat. Add the broccoli, carrots, onion, and garlic, and sauté until the vegetables begin to soften.
2. Add the chicken and 1 tablespoon of the teriyaki sauce. When the chicken begins to brown, add the second tablespoon of sauce. Cook for an additional 10 to 15 minutes, or until the chicken is cooked through (no pink shows in the middle). Serve immediately.

NUTRITION PER SERVING
Calories 210 • Fat 3 g • Fiber 5 g • Protein 31 g • Carbohydrates 15 g

# beth's chicken and broccoli bake

MAKES 4 SERVINGS

This baked dish works well for almost every dinner mood.

**Cooking spray**
**8 ounces corkscrew pasta**
**4 cups frozen broccoli**
**1 (10.75-ounce) can reduced-fat cream of chicken soup**
**1 boneless, skinless chicken breast half, cooked and chopped**
**1 teaspoon salt**

1. Preheat the oven to 350°F. Lightly coat an 8-inch-square casserole dish with cooking spray.
2. Bring a large pot of water to a boil. Salt the water and add the pasta; cook according to the package directions. Add the broccoli to the pasta water for the final 2 minutes of cooking. Drain and set aside.
3. Stir together the cream of chicken soup, chicken, and salt in a large bowl.
4. Stir the noodles and broccoli into the chicken mixture. Spoon the mixture into the prepared casserole dish and bake for 20 to 30 minutes, or until hot and bubbly.

NUTRITION PER SERVING

Calories 340 • Fat 6 g • Fiber 4 g • Protein 17 g • Carbohydrates 52 g

# flamin' poultry

MAKES 2 SERVINGS

The flamin' part depends on how generous you are with the hot sauce.

**2 teaspoons butter**
**¼ cup hot sauce**
**2 boneless, skinless chicken breast halves, cut into bite-size pieces**

1. Melt the butter in a skillet over medium heat. Add the hot sauce and mix.
2. Add the chicken, stir to coat, and cover. Cook for about 10 minutes, or until the chicken is cooked through (no pink shows in the middle).

NUTRITION PER SERVING

Calories 170 • Fat 5 g • Fiber 0 g • Protein 27 g • Carbohydrates 0 g

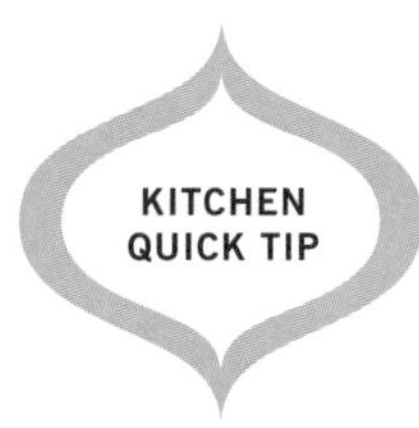


## 7 quick sautés for chicken strips

- Sauté with salsa or hot sauce and use the mixture as a tortilla filling.
- For fried chicken, coat chicken in egg, roll in flour, salt, and pepper, and sauté in canola oil.
- Sauté chicken in a blend of white vinegar, soy sauce, ginger, and garlic for a quick teriyaki.
- Add some vegetables and call it a stir-fry.
- For a hot spinach salad, sauté chicken with mushrooms, onions, and garlic, and serve on a bed of fresh spinach.
- If you have leftover rice, sauté chicken with chopped tomato, onion, garlic, white wine, and rosemary; add rice when the chicken is cooked, heat through, and serve.
- Sauté chicken with salt and pepper. Serve it on a roll with lettuce and tomato for a hot chicken sandwich.

# crispy cracker chicken

MAKES 2 SERVINGS

You can make a fantastic sandwich with these chicken breasts and some sliced tomato.

**1 egg**
**½ cup crushed low-fat wheat crackers, such as Wheat Thins**
**½ cup grated Parmesan cheese**
**2 boneless, skinless chicken breast halves**

1. Preheat the oven to 350°F.
2. Separate the white of the egg into a small bowl or dish, and beat well. Discard the yolk. In a separate dish, mix the crushed crackers and Parmesan.
3. Rinse and pat dry the chicken breasts. Coat with first the egg white and then the cracker mixture.
4. Place the chicken in a pan and bake for about 35 minutes, until the chicken is cooked through (no pink shows in the middle) and the cracker coating is crispy.

NUTRITION PER SERVING

Calories 320 • Fat 12 g • Fiber 0 g • Protein 39 g • Carbohydrates 11 g

# slow-cooked barbecue chicken

MAKES 4 TO 6 SERVINGS

Barbecue without any fuss! It's a real treat to come in the door at the end of a long day, smell the delicious barbecue, and realize you have a hot meal waiting for you without any effort.

**1 whole chicken**
**Salt and freshly ground black pepper**
**1 (8-ounce) bottle of your favorite barbecue sauce**

Rinse the chicken and pat dry with paper towels. Place it in a slow cooker and sprinkle with salt and pepper. Pour a bottle of your favorite barbecue sauce over it, cover, and cook on the low setting for 8 to 10 hours.

NUTRITION PER SERVING

Calories 140 • Fat 3.5 g • Fiber 0 g • Protein 23 g • Carbohydrates 4 g

# balsamic mustard chicken with potatoes

MAKES 4 SERVINGS

Impressive enough for company and guaranteed to please every palate.

- **3 tablespoons Dijon mustard**
- **¼ cup balsamic vinegar**
- **2 tablespoons red wine vinegar**
- **3 tablespoons finely chopped onion**
- **2 garlic cloves, minced**
- **2 tablespoons canola oil**
- **4 boneless, skinless chicken breast halves, cut into 1-inch strips**
- **2 medium red potatoes, peeled and very thinly sliced**
- **½ cup low-sodium chicken broth**

1. Combine the mustard, vinegars, onion, garlic, and 1 tablespoon of the oil in a shallow dish or ziplock bag. Add the chicken and marinate in the refrigerator for 30 minutes.
2. Heat the remaining 1 tablespoon of oil in a skillet over medium heat. Add the potato slices and cook until slightly crisp.
3. Add the chicken and marinade to the pan. Bring to a boil, reduce heat, and simmer for 10 to 15 minutes, until the chicken is cooked through (no pink shows in the middle) and the potatoes are soft.
4. Add the broth and simmer for an additional 5 minutes, until the sauce reaches the desired consistency. Serve hot.

NUTRITION PER SERVING

Calories 310 • Fat 9 g • Fiber 2 g • Protein 30 g • Carbohydrates 23 g

# garlicky olive chicken

MAKES 4 SERVINGS

Buy bone-in chicken pieces if you don't want to cut up a chicken.

- **1 cup black California olives, pitted and halved**
- **1 whole chicken, cut into 6 pieces**
- **3 garlic cloves, peeled and halved**
- **½ cup chopped fresh flat-leaf parsley**
- **2 tablespoons grated lemon zest**
- **8 ounces cherry tomatoes (halve the tomatoes if they're large)**
- **2 tablespoons extra-virgin olive oil**
- **Salt and freshly ground black pepper**

1. Preheat the oven to 400°F. If the olives are very salty, soak them in cold water for 5 minutes and then drain.

2. Place the chicken pieces in a baking dish in a single layer, skin side up. Tuck a piece of garlic under each chicken piece. In a separate bowl mix together the olives, parsley, lemon zest, tomatoes, olive oil, and salt and pepper to taste. Spoon the mixture evenly over the chicken.

3. Bake for 45 to 55 minutes, uncovered, until the chicken is golden and cooked through. Place the chicken on serving plates and drizzle the contents of the pan, including the juices, over the chicken.

NUTRITION PER SERVING

Calories 320 • Fat 16 g • Fiber 2 g • Protein 36 g • Carbohydrates 6 g

# chicken with olives and tomatoes

MAKES 4 SERVINGS

Serve this recipe on a bed of hot rice.

- **½ tablespoon extra-virgin olive oil**
- **4 boneless, skinless chicken breast halves**
- **1 large yellow onion, finely chopped**
- **2 tablespoons red wine vinegar**
- **2 large tomatoes, chopped**
- **⅔ cup pitted and sliced black olives**
- **Salt and freshly ground black pepper**

1. Heat the oil in a large skillet over medium heat. Add the chicken, cover, and cook for 10 to 15 minutes, until the chicken is cooked through (no pink shows in the middle). Remove the chicken from the pan and set aside.
2. Add the onion, vinegar, tomatoes, and olives to the pan with the chicken juice. Bring to a simmer over medium heat and cook for 5 minutes. Return the chicken to the pan and cook until heated through. Season with salt and pepper to taste and serve hot.

NUTRITION PER SERVING

Calories 200 • Fat 6 g • Fiber 2 g • Protein 29 g • Carbohydrates 8 g

# chicken kabobs

MAKES 4 SERVINGS

Resusable metal skewers or disposable bamboo skewers are both fine for this recipe. Soak bamboo skewers in water for at least 30 minutes before using.

**4 boneless, skinless chicken breast halves, cut into bite-size pieces**
**¾ cup teriyaki marinade (see page 249 for our recipe)**
**8 cherry tomatoes**
**1 yellow onion, cut into large wedges**
**1 green bell pepper, seeded and cut into large chunks**
**8 mushrooms, wiped clean**

1. Marinate the chicken in the teriyaki sauce for 30 minutes in the refrigerator.
2. Preheat the grill or broiler.
3. Thread the chicken, tomatoes, onion, green pepper, and mushrooms onto skewers, alternating ingredients.
4. Over a red-hot grill or under the broiler, cook the kabobs for 10 to 15 minutes, until the chicken is cooked through (no pink shows in the middle). Serve on or off the skewer over a bed of rice.

NUTRITION PER SERVING

Calories 240 • Fat 1.5 g • Fiber 2 g • Protein 31 g • Carbohydrates 23 g

# chicken curry

MAKES 2 SERVINGS

A lot of curry recipes are complicated, but this one is both easy and delicious.

**¼ cup all-purpose flour**
**½ tablespoon sugar**
**2 teaspoons curry powder**
**¼ teaspoon ground ginger**
**1 tablespoon butter**
**¼ cup diced onion**
**½ cup chicken broth**
**½ cup milk**
**1½ teaspoons lemon juice**
**1 boneless, skinless chicken breast half, cooked and cubed**
**Vegetables of choice, such as carrots, peas, or mushrooms**
**Cooked rice**

1. Mix together the flour, sugar, curry powder, and ginger in a small bowl.
2. Melt the butter in a large skillet over medium heat. Add the onion and sauté until tender. Add the flour mixture and cook for 2 minutes. Slowly pour in the chicken broth and milk. Simmer until thick and bubbly, stirring often.
3. Stir in the lemon juice, chicken, and vegetables; cook 5 minutes longer, or until the vegetables are tender. Serve over hot rice.

NUTRITION PER SERVING

Calories 230 • Fat 7 g • Fiber 1 g • Protein 19 g • Carbohydrates 22 g

## cobb burger

MAKES 4 SERVINGS

This is a healthier, more delicious version of the standard hamburger. Round out the meal with Sweet Potato Fries (page 246).

**1 pound ground chicken**
**1 onion, minced**
**¼ cup crumbled blue cheese**
**Salt and freshly ground black pepper**
**1 tablespoon vegetable oil**
**8 strips lean bacon**
**1 avocado**
**¼ cup low-fat mayonnaise**
**Lettuce and sliced tomato for garnish**
**4 kaiser rolls**

1. Combine the chicken, onion, and blue cheese. Season with salt and pepper. Form the mixture into 4 patties.
2. Heat the oil in a skillet over medium to medium-high heat. Pan-fry the patties in the skillet for 4 to 5 minutes on each side, until the juices run clear.
3. While the patties are cooking, cook the bacon in a separate pan until it's crisp. Drain the bacon on a paper towel.
4. Dice the avocado and combine with the mayonnaise.
5. To assemble the burgers, place a patty on the bottom half of each kaiser roll. Top with the bacon, some lettuce, a slice of tomato, and a spoonful of the avocado mixture. Put the top part of the roll on each burger and enjoy!

NUTRITION PER SERVING

Calories 470 • Fat 18 g • Fiber 3 g • Protein 35 g • Carbohydrates 30 g

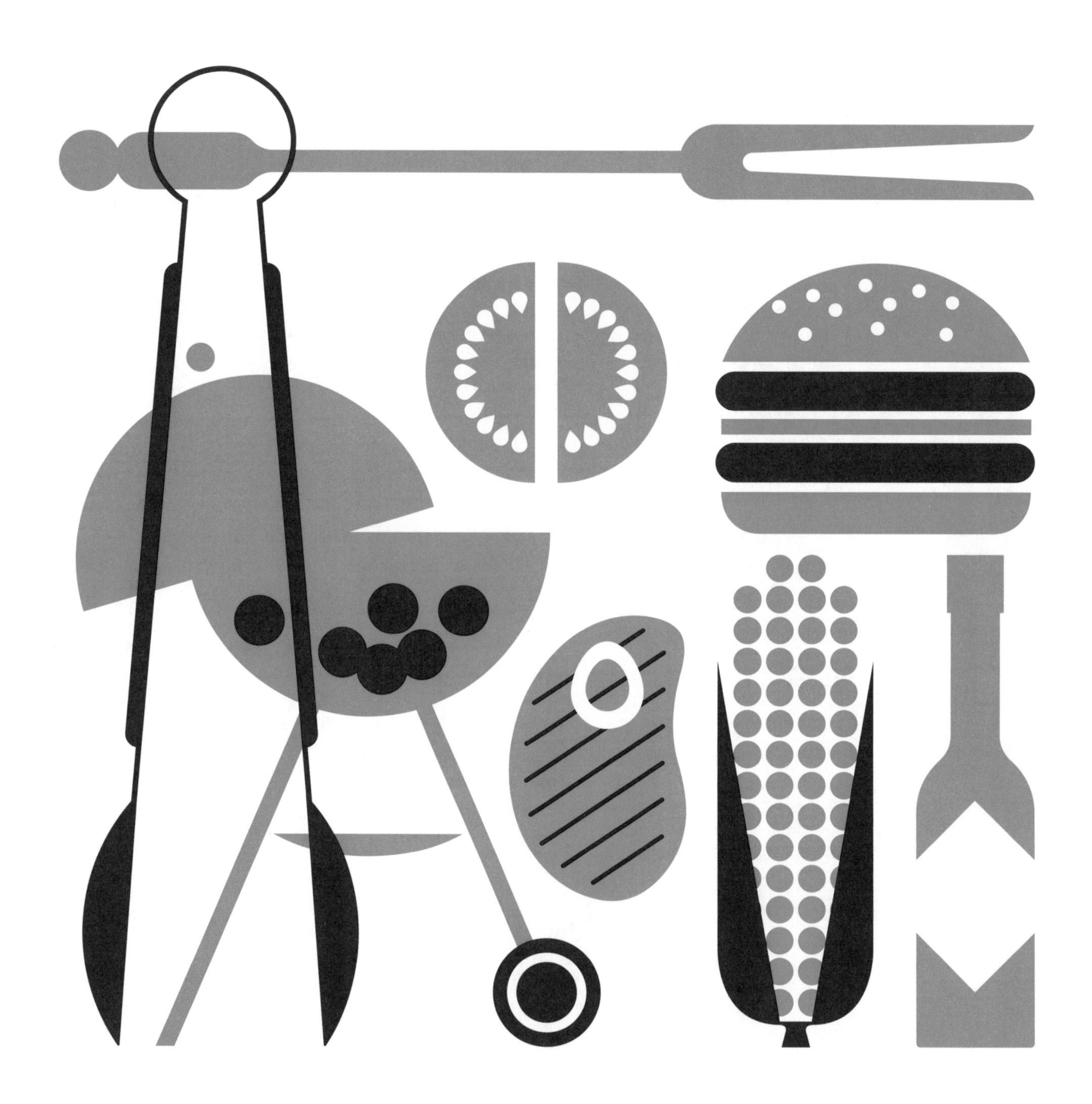

# chapter 9

## dishes for meat lovers

We must admit that dining-hall food did frighten us away from meat for a brief time, but we've realized that when you're in control of buying, preparing, and cooking meat, it offers great variety. Barbecuing is fun, marinating is effortless, and there is an endless variety of seasonings and herbs to use.

This chapter deals with non-chicken meats: beef, pork, and turkey. It is important to make sure that your cut or roast is fresh when you buy it. Check the date, look for discoloration (green = bad), and smell your purchase. When cooking any kind of meat, take heed of the "Handling Meats" cautions listed on page 20. As you probably know, raw meat can contain harmful bacteria, so all utensils, countertops, pans, bowls, and everything else that comes in contact with the raw meat, even the kitchen sink, should be carefully cleaned with soap and hot water. While this is a serious issue, don't let it scare you away. If you are careful and clean properly, your meal will be fine. Enjoy our recommendations and have fun creating your own.

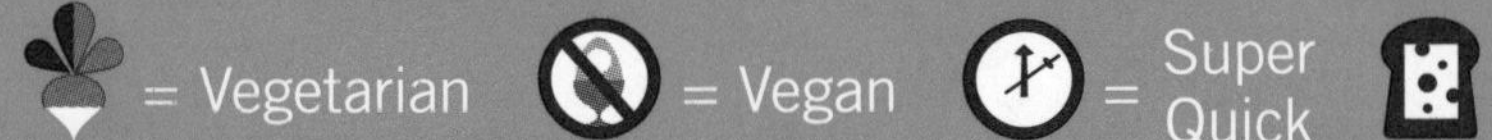
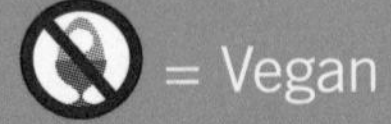
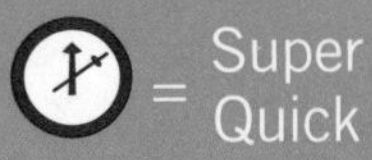
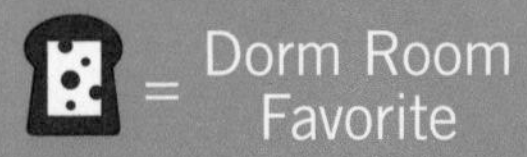

= Vegetarian = Vegan = Super Quick = Dorm Room Favorite

# beef 'n' barley dinner

MAKES 6 SERVINGS

This hearty meal is a delicious, quick, easy, and cheap way to feed a crowd! You can add vegetables, too — try carrots, mushrooms, squash, or whatever else you have on hand.

**1 pound lean ground beef**
**1 onion, diced**
**2 teaspoons no-salt herb seasoning**
**1 (11-ounce) box quick-cooking barley**
**1 cup shredded cheddar cheese**

1. Combine the beef, onion, and seasoning in a skillet over medium heat. Cook, stirring often, until the beef is browned and crumbled into small pieces. Drain the grease from the skillet.
2. While the beef mixture is cooking, cook the barley according to the package directions.
3. Stir the beef mixture into the barley. Add the cheese, mix well, and serve immediately.

NUTRITION PER SERVING

Calories 310 • Fat 5 g • Fiber 8 g • Protein 25 g • Carbohydrates 43 g

# beer beef stew

MAKES 4 SERVINGS

This is great alone or over a bed of hot cooked rice. If the stew seems too dry to your taste, you can add some extra beef broth.

**1 teaspoon extra-virgin olive oil**
**1 pound chuck steak, cut into 1-inch cubes**
**½ cup chopped onion**
**½ cup chopped green bell pepper**
**1½ (12-ounce) bottles beer**
**½ teaspoon dried oregano**
**1 teaspoon dried basil**
**Salt and freshly ground black pepper**
**1 low-sodium beef bouillon cube**
**1¼ cups water**
**2 tablespoons all-purpose flour**
**½ cup chopped carrots**
**1 cup chopped potatoes**

1 Heat the oil in a large pot over medium heat. Add the steak and sauté until browned. Add the onion and green pepper, reduce heat, cover, and cook for 5 minutes.

2 Add the beer. Season with the oregano, basil, and salt and pepper to taste. Bring to a boil; stir in the bouillon cube and 1 cup of the water. Bring back to a boil, then reduce the heat, cover, and simmer, stirring occasionally, for 1 hour or until the beef is very tender.

3 Whisk the flour into the remaining ¼ cup of water and stir the mixture into the stew (this will prevent the flour from getting lumpy when it is added). Stir the carrots and potatoes into the stew. Cover and simmer, stirring occasionally, for 40 minutes, or until the vegetables are tender.

NUTRITION PER SERVING

Calories 330 • Fat 13 g • Fiber 2 g • Protein 24 g • Carbohydrates 19 g

# beef stir-fry

MAKES 4 SERVINGS

Serve this stir-fry alone or with sticky rice or couscous. It's also good with chicken instead of beef, or different vegetables instead of broccoli. Use whatever's in the refrigerator — it's all good.

- **⅔ cup low-sodium soy sauce**
- **2 scallions, sliced**
- **Freshly ground black pepper**
- **2 teaspoons packed brown sugar**
- **1½ pounds top round or flank steak, thinly sliced against the grain**
- **1½ tablespoons vegetable oil**
- **1 teaspoon sesame oil**
- **1 medium onion, chopped**
- **4 cups chopped broccoli**

1. Combine the soy sauce, scallions, pepper, and sugar in a large bowl. Add the beef, stir well, and marinate for 10 minutes.
2. Heat the vegetable oil and sesame oil in a large skillet over medium heat. Add the beef, marinade, onion, and broccoli, and sauté until the meat is cooked to your liking, stirring occasionally. Add a little water if there's not enough liquid in the pan.

NUTRITION PER SERVING

Calories 470 • Fat 21 g • Fiber 5 g • Protein 53 g • Carbohydrates 16 g

# ginger-garlic beef stir-fry

MAKES 2 SERVINGS

This is a variation of the Beef Stir-Fry on page 208; it's sweeter and is flavored with garlic and ginger rather than onion. Though you can serve it on its own, it goes well with rice.

**½ pound top round or flank steak, thinly sliced against the grain**
**3 garlic cloves, minced**
**3 tablespoons freshly grated ginger**
**5 tablespoons low-sodium soy sauce**
**1 good-size head broccoli (or 1 package frozen broccoli, thawed)**
**3 tablespoons packed brown sugar (or less, if you prefer a less sweet dish)**
**3 tablespoons oyster sauce**
**1 tablespoon vegetable oil**

1. Combine the beef, garlic, and ginger in a small bowl. Add 3 tablespoons of the soy sauce, stir well, and marinate for at least 10 minutes or up to 1 hour.
2. Chop the broccoli into small florets.
3. Mix together the sugar, oyster sauce, and the remaining 2 tablespoons of soy sauce in a small bowl.
4. Heat the oil in a wok or skillet over medium-high heat. When the oil begins to sizzle, add the beef and its marinade. Sauté the beef, stirring often, until browned.
5. Add the broccoli and cook for 3 to 4 minutes, until tender.
6. Pour in the soy sauce mixture. Continue to cook, stirring often, until the sauce is hot. Serve hot.

**NUTRITION PER SERVING**
Calories 450 • Fat 17 g • Fiber 5 g • Protein 39 g • Carbohydrates 37 g

# beef burritos

MAKES 4 SERVINGS

Make up extra burritos, wrap tightly in plastic wrap, and freeze for quick meals on busy days.

**1 pound lean ground beef**
**1 teaspoon cayenne pepper**
**1 teaspoon chili powder**
**1 teaspoon hot sauce**
**8 flour tortillas**
**1 tomato, diced**
**Grilled vegetables of your choice, diced (optional)**
**½ cup chopped lettuce**
**Salsa**

1. Heat a skillet over medium-high heat. Add the beef, cayenne, chili powder, and hot sauce and cook until the beef is browned, stirring to break up the beef.

2. Serve the beef, tortillas, tomato, grilled vegetables, if using, lettuce, and salsa on separate plates, buffet-style. To make a burrito, place a couple of spoonfuls of ingredients in the center of a tortilla. Fold 1 edge up to make a bottom lip over the filling, then fold the sides in to overlap in the center, making a secure basket for the filling.

NUTRITION PER SERVING

Calories 480 • Fat 20 g • Fiber 3 g • Protein 28 g • Carbohydrates 35 g

# tacos

MAKES 4 SERVINGS

This recipe includes the basics of any good taco. However, for more variety and a healthier palette, consider adding to the buffet table grilled or roasted vegetables of all sorts — green and red peppers, onions, zucchini, and mushrooms are good choices. It's a great way to use up leftover vegetables, as well as a great excuse for making extra vegetables the night before.

**1 pound lean ground beef**
**8 taco shells**
**1 tomato, diced**
**½ cup chopped lettuce**
**Salsa**
**Hot sauce**

1. Heat a nonstick skillet over medium-high heat. Add the beef and cook until browned, stirring to break up the beef.
2. Transfer the beef to a plate. Serve buffet-style with the taco shells, tomato, lettuce, salsa, and hot sauce.

NUTRITION PER SERVING
Calories 360 • Fat 19 g • Fiber 2 g • Protein 25 g • Carbohydrates 20 g

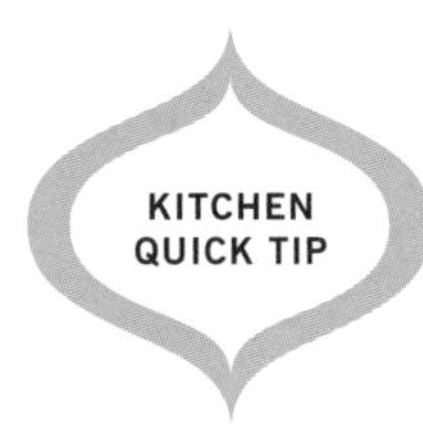


## keep it lean

The nutritional analyses for the tacos and burritos assume that the fat from the ground beef stays with the meat as it is cooked and served. To cut down on fat, drain the skillet after cooking, and pat the cooked ground beef with a paper towel to absorb excess grease. You won't be able to get rid of all of it, but you can make a sizable dent.

# turkey burgers

MAKES 4 SERVINGS

You can cook the burgers two at a time, depending on how big your pan is. To make sure that they're fully cooked, cut one burger open to its middle. If it's still pink, keep cooking.

**1½ pounds lean ground turkey**
**¼ cup whole-wheat breadcrumbs**
**2 garlic cloves, minced**
**1 teaspoon hot sauce (optional)**
**Freshly ground black pepper**
**1 teaspoon extra-virgin olive oil**

1. Combine the turkey, breadcrumbs, garlic, hot sauce, if using, and a pinch of pepper in a large bowl, and mix well with your hands. Form the mixture into 4 patties.
2. Heat the oil in a nonstick skillet over medium heat. Cook the burgers in the oil for 5 minutes per side, or until done (no pink shows in the middle). Be careful when flipping the burgers; turkey does not hold together as well as beef burgers do.

NUTRITION PER SERVING
Calories 260 • Fat 12 g • Fiber 0 g • Protein 34 g • Carbohydrates 5 g

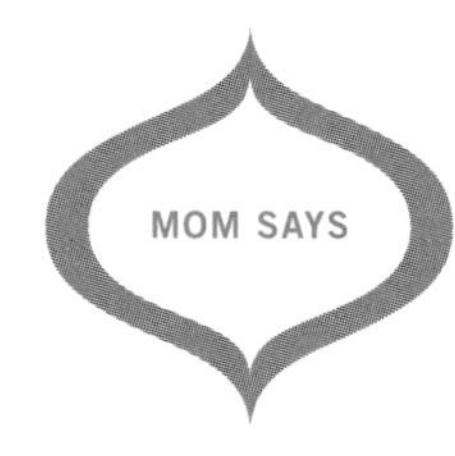


## burger tips

- In most recipes, ground turkey is a great substitute for ground beef. Lean ground turkey usually contains less fat than lean ground beef.
- We didn't use egg in our burger recipes because we think it adds unnecessary bad stuff (like cholesterol). But that comes with a price tag: these burgers may crumble a little if you're not careful with them. If you want burgers that are easier to handle and you don't mind a little extra cholesterol, try adding an egg or two (or just their whites) to these recipes.

# stan's southern burgers

MAKES 4 SERVINGS

The mushrooms and salsa are an unexpected, but delicious, combination in these burgers.

**1¼ pounds lean ground beef**
**¼ cup whole-wheat breadcrumbs**
**2 medium mushrooms, wiped clean and diced**
**1 tablespoon salsa**
**1 teaspoon hot sauce**

1. Preheat the grill.
2. Combine all of the ingredients in a large bowl and mix thoroughly with your hands. Form the mixture into 4 patties.
3. Grill the patties for about 4 minutes per side for medium, or until done to your satisfaction.

NUTRITION PER SERVING
Calories 190 • Fat 6 g • Fiber 0 g • Protein 29 g • Carbohydrates 5 g

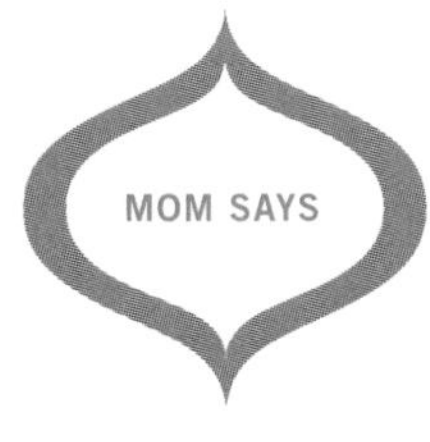


## more burger tips

- When freezing leftover raw ground beef, mold it into hamburger patties first. You can then defrost only the amount you need for the particular meal you will be preparing.
- To make your own breadcrumbs, toast a slice of stale bread, then toss it in the blender for a few seconds. No blender? Just use a knife to scrape the toast into crumbs.

# steak à l'orange

MAKES 4 SERVINGS

Add a baked potato and a salad for the full steak-house experience.

**2 oranges (preferably organic)**
**2 teaspoons extra-virgin olive oil**
**1 teaspoon chili powder**
**4 (8-ounce) beefsteaks**
**Salt and freshly ground black pepper**

1. Preheat the grill or broiler.
2. Zest the oranges with a grater or microplane. Combine the zest with the oil and chili powder. Mix well. Spread the oil mixture evenly over both sides of each steak.
3. Grill or broil the steaks for 5 minutes on each side for medium, or to desired doneness.
4. Squeeze some orange juice over the top of each steak. Season to taste with salt and pepper.

NUTRITION PER SERVING
Calories 480 • Fat 21 g • Fiber 2 g • Protein 63 g • Carbohydrates 8 g

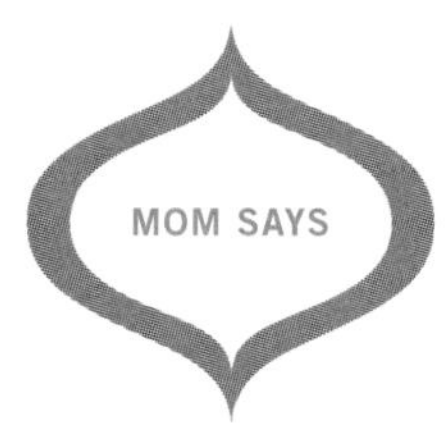


## using the whole lemon

When a recipe calls for the zest and the juice of a lemon (or an orange or lime), zest the fruit first with a grater or microplane. Then you can cut the fruit in half and squeeze out the juice. If you juice the lemon first, it's difficult to zest the crushed fruit.

# flank steak

MAKES 4 SERVINGS

The simple marinade used here is also very tasty with chicken or salmon.

**⅔ cup low-sodium soy sauce**
**¼ cup packed brown sugar**
**2 teaspoons freshly grated ginger**
**1½ pounds flank steak**

1. Combine the soy sauce, sugar, and ginger in a shallow dish or ziplock bag. Marinate the steak in the mixture for at least 3 hours in the refrigerator.
2. Preheat the broiler.
3. Remove the steak from the marinade and broil for about 5 minutes per side, until done to your satisfaction. For a more intense flavor, pan-cook the steak in the marinade.

NUTRITION PER SERVING

Calories 400 • Fat 14 g • Fiber 0 g • Protein 50 g • Carbohydrates 17 g

# uncle j's meat loaf

MAKES 4 SERVINGS

Make a little extra of this recipe. It tastes good cold and makes a great sandwich that will really fill you up. It's a good way to plan ahead if you know that you have a hectic week coming up.

**¼ cup skim milk**
**1 slice whole-grain bread**
**¾ pound lean ground beef**
**½ onion, chopped**
**1 egg, beaten**
**¼ cup chopped fresh parsley**
**¼ cup ketchup**
**½ teaspoon hot sauce**
**Salt and freshly ground black pepper**

1. Preheat the oven to 350°F.

2. Pour the milk into a medium bowl and place the bread on top. When the bread has absorbed most of the milk (3 to 4 minutes), add the beef, onion, egg, parsley, ketchup, hot sauce, and pinches of salt and pepper. Mix with your hands until no chunks of bread are visible.

3. Pat the mixture into a loaf shape in a small casserole or baking dish and bake for 1 hour, or until cooked through (no pink shows in the middle).

4. Remove the loaf from the oven and cool for 10 minutes. Carefully drain the liquid from the dish, making sure not to lose the loaf to the sink. Serve in slices.

NUTRITION PER SERVING

Calories 280 • Fat 16 g • Fiber 1 g • Protein 20 g • Carbohydrates 9 g

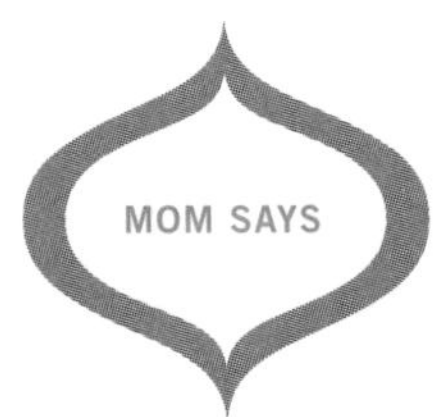


## adding fiber

Adding oats to a meat loaf provides greater fiber content and doesn't affect the flavor. Try adding a handful or two to each loaf.

# mexican lasagna

MAKES 6 SERVINGS

This one will take a little extra time, but it's worth it.

- 2 teaspoons extra-virgin olive oil
- 1 large onion, chopped
- ½ green bell pepper, seeded and chopped
- 3 garlic cloves, minced
- 1¼ pounds lean ground beef
- 2 tablespoons chopped jalapeño pepper
- 2 cups tomato sauce
- 1½ cups low-sodium beef broth
- Salt
- 1 tablespoon all-purpose flour
- 3 tablespoons finely chopped fresh cilantro (optional)
- 2 cups shredded low-fat cheddar cheese
- 6 small flour tortillas, cut into three strips each

1. Preheat the oven to 350°F.
2. Heat the oil in a large skillet over medium heat. Add the onion and green pepper and sauté until the onion is translucent. Add the garlic and cook an additional 2 minutes. Add the beef and cook until browned, stirring to break up the beef. Stir in the jalapeño, tomato sauce, ¾ cup of the beef broth, and a pinch of salt.
3. In a bowl, whisk the flour into the remaining ¾ cup of beef broth. Add the flour mixture to the beef mixture, bring to a boil, and then reduce the heat and simmer until the sauce thickens. Remove from the heat, add the cilantro, if using, and stir well.
4. Fill a casserole dish with the sauce, cheese, and tortilla strips in alternating layers, beginning with a thin sauce layer and ending with a cheese layer. Bake for 15 to 20 minutes or until heated through.

NUTRITION PER SERVING

Calories 460 • Fat 26 g • Fiber 3 g • Protein 33 g • Carbohydrates 26 g

# real sloppy sloppy joe

MAKES 4 SERVINGS

Soy-based ground beef substitutes also make tasty Sloppy Joes if you would like a vegetarian version.

- **1½ pounds lean ground beef**
- **½ yellow onion, finely chopped**
- **1 garlic clove, minced**
- **½ cup ketchup**
- **¼ cup crushed tomatoes (or tomato sauce)**
- **1 tablespoon red wine vinegar**
- **2 tablespoons Worcestershire sauce**
- **2 teaspoons hot sauce**
- **Salt and freshly ground black pepper**
- **4 hamburger buns**

1. Heat a nonstick skillet over medium heat. Add the beef, onion, and garlic, and cook until the beef is browned, stirring to break up the beef. Drain the excess fat from the skillet.
2. Add the ketchup, crushed tomatoes, vinegar, Worcestershire, hot sauce, and salt and pepper to taste to the skillet. Stir well, heat to a simmer, and simmer for 5 minutes.
3. While the beef mixture simmers, toast the hamburger buns.
4. Arrange the buns open on plates. Ladle a healthy portion of the beef mixture over each and serve immediately.

NUTRITION PER SERVING

Calories 530 • Fat 30 g • Fiber 1 g • Protein 38 g • Carbohydrates 33 g

# slow-cooked shredded italian beef

MAKES 6 SERVINGS

Use this savory beef to make sandwiches with lettuce, tomato, onion, or whatever other fresh vegetables you like.

**1 (3–4 pound) beef round roast**
**2 packages dry Italian dressing mix**
**1–1½ (12-ounce) bottles beer**

1. Trim any visible fat from the roast; place it in a slow cooker. Sprinkle with dry Italian dressing and pour in 1 bottle of beer. Cover and cook on the low setting for 6 to 8 hours. Check the meat every couple of hours; if the slow cooker begins to run low on liquid, add the other half-bottle of beer.
2. When the roast is fully cooked and falling apart, use 2 forks to shred it. Enjoy warm or cold. Don't forget to store the leftovers in the refrigerator.

NUTRITION PER SERVING
Calories 630 • Fat 23 g • Fiber 0 g • Protein 89 g • Carbohydrates 5 g

# chili con carne

MAKES 6 SERVINGS

A simple recipe that will satisfy your taste for a spicy, warming bowl of chili.

**1 pound lean ground beef**
**1 teaspoon extra-virgin olive oil**
**½ cup chopped onion**
**2 garlic cloves, minced**
**2 (15-ounce) cans chopped tomatoes, drained**
**2 (15-ounce) cans kidney beans, rinsed and drained**
**2 tablespoons chili powder**
**1 tablespoon sugar**
**Pinch of salt**
**Pinch of freshly ground black pepper**
**Small pinch of nutmeg**
**1 bay leaf**

1 Heat a skillet over medium heat. Add the beef and cook until browned, stirring to break up the beef. Drain the fat from the skillet.

2 While the beef is browning, heat the oil in a large pot over medium heat. Add the onion and garlic and sauté for 4 to 6 minutes, until the onion is tender. Add the tomatoes, beans, chili powder, sugar, salt and pepper, nutmeg, and bay leaf, and stir well.

3 Add the beef to the chili. Bring to a simmer and cook, covered, for 1½ hours. Discard the bay leaf.

NUTRITION PER SERVING

Calories 270 • Fat 5 g • Fiber 10 g • Protein 24 g • Carbohydrates 34 g

# beef stroganoff

MAKES 4 SERVINGS

An old-fashioned dinner party meal that still tastes great today.

**8 ounces egg noodles**
**1¼ pounds top round beef, thinly sliced against the grain**
**¼ cup sliced onions**
**1 tablespoon all-purpose flour**
**1 garlic clove, minced**
**8 fresh mushrooms, wiped clean and sliced**
**½ cup low-sodium chicken broth**
**½ cup nonfat sour cream**
**Salt and freshly ground black pepper**
**Chopped fresh parsley**

1. Bring a pot of water to a boil. Salt the water and add the noodles; cook according to the package directions. Drain and set aside.
2. While the noodles are cooking, heat a skillet over medium heat. Add the beef and onions. As the beef begins to brown, stir in the flour so that it coats the beef. Stir in the garlic, mushrooms, chicken broth, and sour cream.
3. Cook until the sauce is an even consistency and the mushrooms are tender. Add salt and pepper to taste. Serve over egg noodles, garnished with plenty of fresh parsley.

NUTRITION PER SERVING

Calories 350 • Fat 5 g • Fiber 2 g • Protein 39 g • Carbohydrates 40 g

# one-pot pot roast

MAKES 8 SERVINGS

This roast cooks for a long time but uses only one pot, which makes cleanup easy. It's a great dish to start before a long afternoon study session — you can enjoy the aromas and look forward to dinner while you work.

**3 tablespoons vegetable oil**
**1 (3–4 pound) chuck roast**
**1 medium yellow onion, sliced**
**2 celery stalks, chopped into 1-inch pieces**
**1 (12-ounce) bottle beer, or 1 cup red wine**
**1 (14.5-ounce) can low-sodium beef broth**
**1 (10.5-ounce) can condensed cream of mushroom soup**
**½ pound new potatoes, washed and halved if large**
**½ pound baby carrots, rinsed**
**1 cup pearl onions, peeled (frozen pearl onions are already peeled and will work fine)**
**Any other vegetables, chopped (optional)**
**Salt and freshly ground black pepper**

1. Heat the oil in a large pot or Dutch oven over medium-high heat. Add the roast to the pot and sear on all sides, making sure that each side is deep golden brown before moving on to the next. Remove the roast from the pot and set aside.
2. Add the onion and celery to the pot and sauté until lightly browned, about 5 minutes.
3. Add the beer to the pot and simmer until reduced by half. Stir often, scraping up any bits of meat that have stuck to the bottom of the pot.
4. Add the broth and soup to the pot and bring to a boil. Reduce the heat to medium, return the meat to the pot, cover, and cook for 3½ to 4 hours, or until the roast is very tender. About 30 minutes before you think the roast will be finished, add the potatoes, carrots, and any other root vegetables you desire to the pot. Ten minutes before the roast is finished, add the pearl onions and any additional vegetables you desire. Season to taste with salt and pepper before serving.

NUTRITION PER SERVING

Calories 420 • Fat 17 g • Fiber 2 g • Protein 45 g • Carbohydrates 16 g

# micki's roast turkey

MAKES 4 TO 6 SERVINGS

Lots of people are scared off by the thought of roasting a turkey. It's actually easy, and it makes great leftovers. For this recipe you'll need a large Dutch-oven-type pot (an ovenproof pot with a lid).

**1 (5–7 pound) bone-in turkey breast**
**1 tablespoon extra-virgin olive oil**
**1 teaspoon salt (kosher salt works best)**
**1 teaspoon freshly ground black pepper**
**1 teaspoon garlic powder**
**1 lemon, halved**
**Sprigs of fresh sage, rosemary, and thyme, tied together in a bundle**
**3 (12-ounce) jars fat-free turkey gravy**
**1 (14.5-ounce) can low-sodium chicken broth**

1. Preheat the oven to 350°F.
2. Rinse the turkey breast and pat dry with paper towels. Rub the exterior of the turkey first with olive oil and then with salt, pepper, and garlic powder. Place the lemon halves and the herb bundle in the turkey cavity.
3. In a large Dutch oven, mix together the turkey gravy and the chicken broth. Place the turkey breast side up in the gravy and cover the pot with the lid.
4. Roast for 1 hour, then check the interior temperature of the breast meat. If the turkey breast came with a pop-up thermometer, it will pop up when the roast is done. If not, you'll need to use a meat thermometer. Insert it into the breast, being sure that its tip doesn't hit the bones; when the interior temperature reaches 170°F, the roast is done. If the roast isn't done after 1 hour, roast for another 20 minutes and then check again.
5. Remove the turkey, take the lemon and herbs out of the cavity, and let the meat rest while you finish the gravy. Place the pot on a stovetop over medium-high heat and cook the gravy for 15 minutes, stirring often, until it thickens.

NUTRITION PER SERVING

Calories 680 • Fat 13 g • Fiber 1 g • Protein 137 g • Carbohydrates 11 g

## beans 'n' franks

 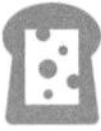

MAKES 2 SERVINGS

A yummy and cheap home-style meal.

**1 (16-ounce) can baked beans**
**3 hot dogs (beef, turkey, chicken, or soy), sliced into rounds**
**2 tablespoons packed brown sugar or maple syrup**

Combine beans, hot dogs, and sugar in a saucepan and heat, stirring often, until hot. You can also combine all ingredients in a microwave-safe bowl, cover, and microwave for about 3 minutes or until heated through. Serve immediately.

NUTRITION PER SERVING
Calories 530 • Fat 23 g • Fiber 14 g • Protein 18 g • Carbohydrates 64 g

## teriyaki pork chops

MAKES 4 SERVINGS

When broiling pork in the oven, place a foil-lined baking sheet on the rack below to catch the juices dripping from the chops.

**1½ cups teriyaki sauce (see page 249 for our recipe)**
**4 boneless pork chops (about 1½ pounds total)**

1. Pour the teriyaki sauce into a shallow dish or ziplock bag. Add the pork chops and marinate in the refrigerator for about 1½ hours.
2. Preheat the broiler or grill.
3. Take the chops out of the marinade and broil or grill for 5 to 8 minutes on each side, or to desired doneness. (When cooked through, the meat will not show any pink in the middle.)

NUTRITION PER SERVING
Calories 400 • Fat 15 g • Fiber 0 g • Protein 30 g • Carbohydrates 33 g

# sweet and sour pork

MAKES 4 SERVINGS

Serve over rice or couscous, making sure to get every last drop of sauce out of the pan and onto your plate.

**1 tablespoon butter**
**1 pound lean pork, cut into small cubes**
**1 medium onion, chopped**
**1½ cups water**
**2 tablespoons packed brown sugar**
**¼ cup raisins**
**1 medium tomato, diced**
**1 sprig fresh rosemary**
**1 tablespoon red wine vinegar**

1. Melt the butter in a saucepan over medium heat. Add the pork and onion and sauté for 5 minutes, until the pork is cooked through (no pink shows).
2. Add the water, sugar, raisins, tomato, and rosemary. Bring to a boil, reduce heat, and simmer, covered, for 10 minutes.
3. Add the vinegar and simmer for 5 minutes longer, stirring often, until the sauce has been reduced by about half. Remove the rosemary sprig and serve.

NUTRITION PER SERVING

Calories 230 • Fat 6 g • Fiber 2 g • Protein 25 g • Carbohydrates 20 g

# pork enchiladas

MAKES 4 SERVINGS

This is an easy make-ahead recipe. You can freeze the uncooked burritos to pull out and bake when you need them.

- **¾ pound lean pork loin**
- **1 can cola**
- **¼ cup packed brown sugar**
- **1 (10-ounce) can green enchilada sauce**
- **1 (8-ounce) box Mexican-style rice (any brand will do; plain rice will also do)**
- **8 whole-wheat tortillas**
- **1 (15-ounce) can black beans, rinsed and drained**
- **1 cup shredded cheddar cheese**

1. Trim any visible veins of fat from the pork. Cut into 1-inch chunks. Place the pork in a slow cooker with the cola. Cover and cook on the low setting for 4 hours, then drain and shred the pork. Mix the shredded pork with the sugar and ¼ cup of the green enchilada sauce.
2. While the pork is still in the slow cooker, prepare the rice according to the package directions.
3. Preheat the oven to 375°F.
4. To make the burritos, place the tortillas on a flat surface. Fill each with a couple of spoonfuls of pork, rice, black beans, and cheese, and top with 1 to 2 tablespoons of enchilada sauce. Wrap them up and place them in a baking pan. Drizzle with more green enchilada sauce and sprinkle with any remaining cheese. Bake for 10 to 20 minutes, or until the cheese has melted.

NUTRITION PER SERVING

Calories 730 • Fat 11 g • Fiber 9 g • Protein 40 g • Carbohydrates 117 g

# ham in cider-raisin sauce

MAKES 4 SERVINGS

The ham is already cooked, so you just want to warm the steak and give it a nice brown surface before serving.

**2 teaspoons extra-virgin olive oil**
**1½ pounds cooked lean ham steak, sliced into 4 even pieces**
**2 tablespoons butter**
**2 tablespoons all-purpose flour**
**1½ cups hard or sweet cider**
**½ cup raisins**
**1 tablespoon sugar**
**1 teaspoon Dijon mustard**

1. Heat the oil in a large skillet over medium heat. Add the ham and cook for about 4 minutes per side, or until browned to your taste. You may want to pat the ham with paper towels to absorb some of the excess grease after it's cooked.
2. Melt the butter in a saucepan over medium heat. Add the flour and cook, stirring constantly, for 2 minutes. Stir in the cider, raisins, sugar, and mustard. Bring to a boil, reduce heat, and simmer for 5 minutes or until thickened.
3. Pour the sauce evenly over the ham steaks and serve.

NUTRITION PER SERVING

Calories 410 • Fat 15 g • Fiber 1 g • Protein 34 g • Carbohydrates 33 g

# slow-cooker bbq ribs

MAKES 3 SERVINGS

These ribs have to cook for a while, but putting the dish together takes only a minute. They are great served with mashed potatoes and green salad.

**1 large sweet onion, sliced**
**6 country-style pork ribs or beef short ribs**
**2 (10-ounce) bottles barbecue sauce**

1. Lay the onion slices on the bottom of the slow cooker. Place the ribs on top of the onions. Pour the bottles of barbecue sauce on top of the ribs and onions.
2. Cover and cook on the low setting for 6 hours or more. The more you cook them, the more tender and falling apart they will be.

NUTRITION PER SERVING

Calories 530 • Fat 9 g • Fiber 2 g • Protein 32 g • Carbohydrates 77 g

# tim's slow-cooked citrus ribs

MAKES 4 SERVINGS

This is a really delicious and easy recipe. Make as many as you can fit in your slow cooker!

**1 rack pork ribs (about 2 pounds)**
**2 tablespoons extra-virgin olive oil**
**Mrs. Dash Original Blend spice mix**
**Seasoned salt**
**Garlic salt**
**Any kind of citrus-based seasoning**
**1 (10-ounce) bottle sweet barbecue sauce**
**3 tablespoons lemon juice**

1. Cut the rack of ribs into 2 pieces so that they will fit easily into your slow cooker. Rub each side of the ribs with olive oil, then season with Mrs. Dash, seasoned salt, garlic salt, and citrus blend.
2. Place the ribs meat side up in the slow cooker and drizzle with barbecue sauce. Pour lemon juice around the outside of the ribs to provide additional liquid in the bottom of the cooker. If you are making more than 1 rack at a time, stack the ribs on top of each other as they are prepared, drizzling the top of each section of ribs with barbecue sauce.
3. Cover and cook on the low setting for 6 to 8 hours, until the meat is falling off of the bones. Enjoy!

NUTRITION PER SERVING

Calories 490 • Fat 20 g • Fiber 0 g • Protein 47 g • Carbohydrates 26 g

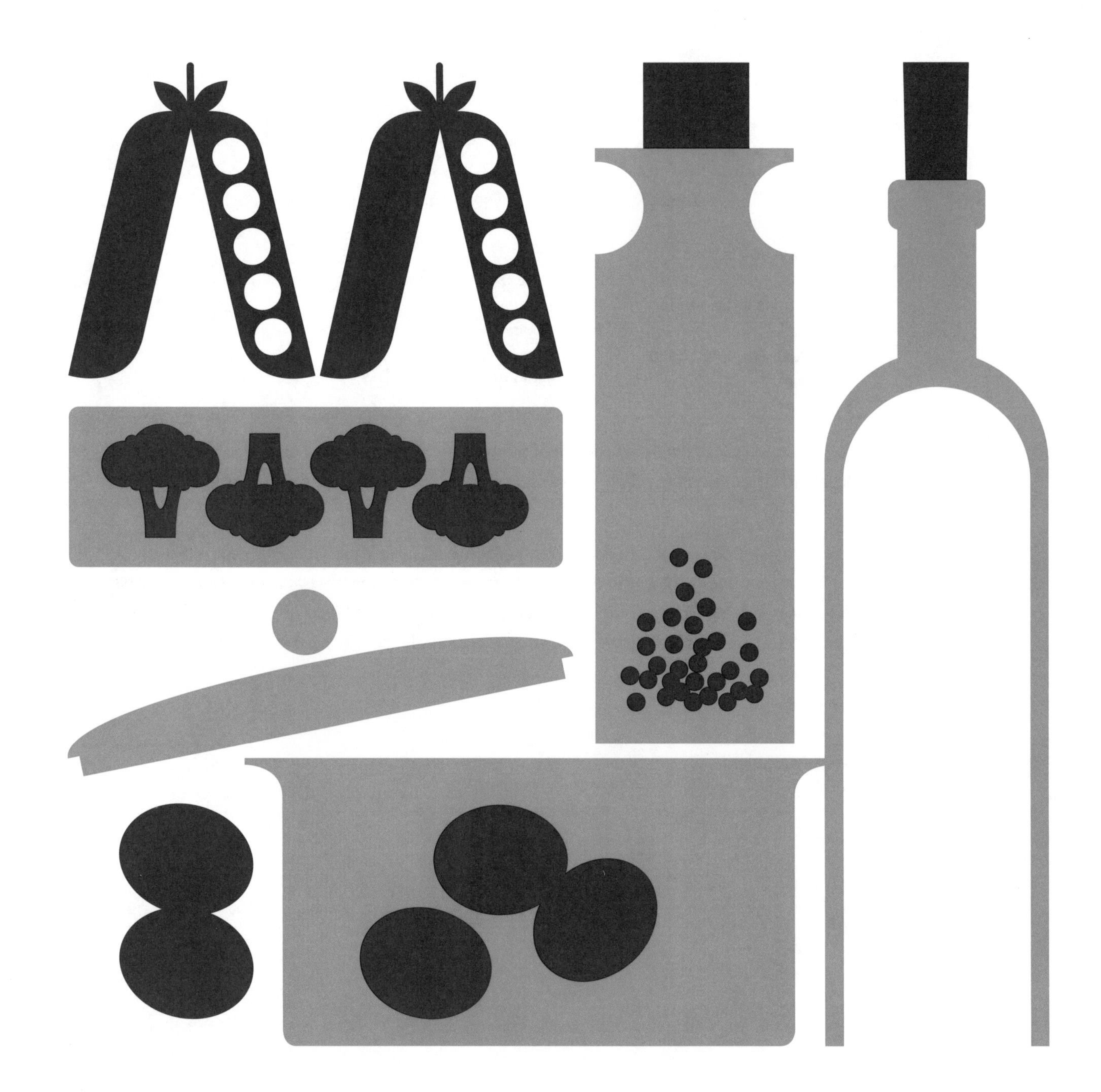

# chapter 10

## side dishes & sauces

Many people, especially students and others with little time or know-how, often think that a single dish will suffice for a full meal. We protest: Side dishes can elevate an everyday meal from good to great. Contrasts in taste and texture, nutritional benefits, and even aesthetics will prove to be worth the small amount of time and energy necessary to prepare these dishes. And your parents will be happy to know that you're eating a well-balanced meal.

Sauces and dressings are also a great way to spice up a side dish or main meal or to give new life to leftovers.

You'll find all of the recipes easy to prepare, but don't feel restricted by our suggestions. There's plenty of room to be creative and discover combinations that suit your own particular tastes.

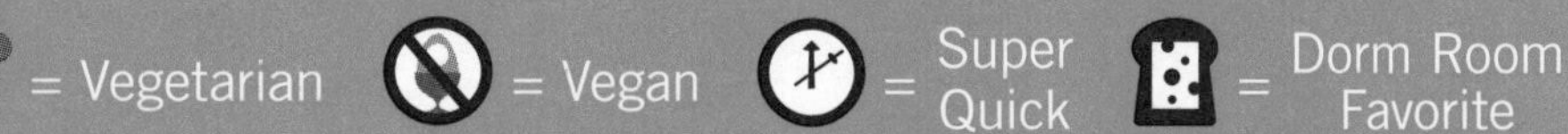


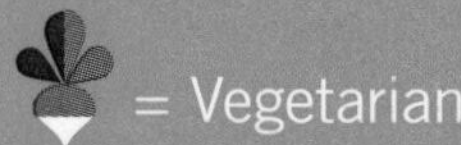

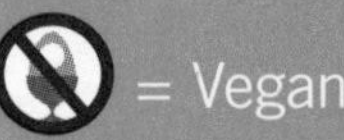

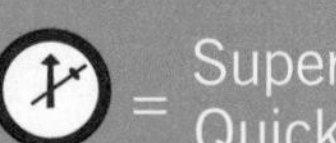

# baked potato

MAKES 1 SERVING

You can also use these instructions for baking a sweet potato.

**1 medium potato**
**Vegetable oil or butter**

1. Preheat the oven to 450°F.
2. Wash the potato and pat dry. Rub oil or butter over the entire skin. Place directly on the oven rack and bake 30 to 45 minutes, until the potato is tender when pierced with a fork. Pierce the skin with a fork about halfway through the baking time to let steam escape and keep the skin from bursting. If you prefer a crispy skin, leave off the oil or butter.

NUTRITION PER SERVING
Calories 220 • Fat 7 g • Fiber 4 g • Protein 4 g • Carbohydrates 37 g

## 6 quick toppings for a baked potato

- Chili
- Salsa and cheese
- Cottage cheese
- Sour cream and chives
- Nonfat refried beans
- Lean ground beef with taco seasoning

# twice-baked potatoes

MAKES 2 SERVINGS

Although this recipe doesn't demand much from the chef, it does require some cooking time, so remember to plan ahead.

**2 medium baking potatoes**
**1 cup fat-free cottage cheese**
**1 hard-boiled egg, finely chopped**
**1 fresh tomato, diced**
**1½ tablespoons Dijon mustard**
**Pinch of salt**
**1½ teaspoons dried dill**
**¾ cup shredded low-fat cheddar cheese**
**¼ teaspoon freshly ground black pepper**

1. Preheat the oven to 400°F.
2. Scrub the potatoes and remove any eyes, then pierce the skin all over with a fork. Bake directly on the oven rack for approximately 1 hour. Remove the potatoes and lower the oven temperature to 325°F.
3. Allow the potatoes to cool until you can handle them comfortably. Slice the potatoes in half lengthwise. Scoop out the insides of the potatoes and place in a mixing bowl, so that you are left with four small potato-skin boats. Set the boats aside.
4. Combine the potato filling with the cottage cheese, egg, tomato, mustard, salt, dill, cheese, and pepper, and mix thoroughly.
5. Place the potato-skin boats on a cookie sheet and overstuff them with the mixture. Bake for 35 minutes, until they're crisp on top. Serve immediately.

NUTRITION PER SERVING

Calories 400 • Fat 11 g • Fiber 6 g • Protein 32 g • Carbohydrates 48 g

# mashed potatoes

MAKES 4 SERVINGS

If you're trying to cut down on fat, omit the butter in this recipe. An easy, low-fat way to spice up mashed potatoes is to add herbs, such as chives or parsley, and nonfat sour cream or plain yogurt.

**2 large potatoes, peeled and quartered**
**2 teaspoons butter**
**1 tablespoon skim milk**
**Salt and freshly ground black pepper**

1. Bring a large pot of water to a boil. Salt the water and add the potatoes; boil until soft, 20 to 30 minutes. Drain.
2. Put the potatoes in a large mixing bowl. Mash them with a fork (or a potato masher, if you're lucky enough to own one). Add the butter, milk, and salt and pepper to taste, and continue mashing until the potatoes reach your desired consistency.

NUTRITION PER SERVING
Calories 160 • Fat 2 g • Fiber 4 g • Protein 4 g • Carbohydrates 32 g

## using up leftovers

Leftover mashed potatoes make delicious potato patties. Just cook the patties in a little butter over medium heat, flipping often, until they're browned to your satisfaction.

# hash browns

MAKES 4 SERVINGS

**2 large potatoes, scrubbed and diced**
**2 teaspoons butter**
**1 small onion, chopped**

1. Bring a medium pot of water to a boil. Salt the water and add the potatoes; cook until tender, about 10 minutes. Drain well.
2. Melt the butter in a large skillet over low heat. Add the potatoes and onion, cover, and cook for 10 minutes. Remove the lid, increase the heat to high, and sauté until the potatoes are browned to your satisfaction.

NUTRITION PER SERVING

Calories 170 • Fat 2 g • Fiber 4 g • Protein 4 g • Carbohydrates 34 g

# applesauce

MAKES 4 SERVINGS

This recipe is also good with a touch of ginger.

**½ cup water**
**4 apples, peeled, cored, and sliced (we recommend McIntosh)**
**½ teaspoon cinnamon**
**Pinch of nutmeg**

1. Bring the water to a boil in a saucepan. Add the apple slices, cover, and cook over low heat for 10 minutes. Turn the heat up to medium and cook, covered, for about 20 minutes more, until the apples are very soft.
2. Remove the pan from the heat and, with a fork or spoon, mash the apples until they reach the desired consistency. Season with cinnamon and nutmeg.

NUTRITION PER SERVING

Calories 100 • Fat 0 g • Fiber 5 g • Protein 0 g • Carbohydrates 25 g

## spaghetti squash with cinnamon

MAKES 4 SERVINGS

**1 large (or 2 small) spaghetti squash, halved and seeded**
**1 tablespoon butter**
**¼ teaspoon salt**
**¼ teaspoon cinnamon**

1. Preheat the oven to 350°F.
2. Place the squash cut side down on a baking sheet. Bake for 45 minutes, or until soft.
3. Scrape out the insides of the squash with a fork, so that the strands begin to separate. Place the pulp in a baking dish. Mix in the butter, salt, and cinnamon. Bake for 15 minutes longer. Serve hot.

NUTRITION PER SERVING
Calories 50 • Fat 3 g • Fiber 2 g • Protein 1 g • Carbohydrates 7 g

## amy's black-eyed peas

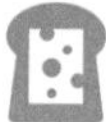

MAKES 4 SERVINGS

**1 cup frozen black-eyed peas**
**1 garlic clove, minced**
**⅓ cup fresh lemon juice**
**2 teaspoons dried or 4 teaspoons chopped fresh mint**
**½ teaspoon salt**

1. Cook the black-eyed peas according to the package directions, making sure they are cooked through. Drain and place in a medium bowl. Cover and refrigerate until chilled.
2. Add the garlic, lemon juice, mint, and salt to the bowl. Mix well and serve cold.

NUTRITION PER SERVING
Calories 45 • Fat 0 g • Fiber 2 g • Protein 3 g • Carbohydrates 10 g

# spaghetti squash marinara

MAKES 4 SERVINGS

When you don't want the carbs that come with a plate of pasta, try this recipe for a change.

**1 large spaghetti squash**
**1 cup marinara sauce**
**½ cup minced fresh parsley**
**½ cup grated Parmesan cheese**
**Salt and freshly ground black pepper**

1. Preheat the oven to 400°F.
2. Use a large, sharp knife to cut the squash in half. Scoop out the seeds and place the squash halves facedown on a lightly greased baking sheet. Bake for 35 to 45 minutes, until the shells are tender enough that you can pierce them easily with a fork.
3. Remove the squash from the oven and lower the oven temperature to 350°F. With a fork, scrape the squash strands from the shells into a large bowl. Mix with the sauce, parsley, and about two-thirds of the cheese. Season with salt and pepper to taste.
4. Place the mixture in a casserole dish, sprinkle the remaining cheese on top, and bake for 15 to 20 minutes, until the squash mixture is heated through and the cheese topping is golden brown.

NUTRITION PER SERVING
Calories 90 • Fat 3.5 g • Fiber 3 g • Protein 11 g • Carbohydrates 11 g

## apple sweet potato

MAKES 4 SERVINGS

**2 teaspoons butter**
**3 tablespoons honey**
**½ tablespoon lemon juice**
**¼ cup sweet or hard cider**
**Salt**
**2 large sweet potatoes, peeled and sliced ¼ inch thick**
**2 medium Granny Smith apples, peeled, cored, and sliced**

1. Preheat the oven to 350°F.
2. Combine the butter, honey, lemon juice, cider, and salt to taste in a small saucepan. Cook over low heat until thoroughly mixed and warm.
3. Arrange the potato and apple slices in a shallow baking dish. Drizzle half of the sauce over the slices. Bake for 45 minutes, basting often with the remaining sauce and any sauce that collects at the bottom of the baking dish.

NUTRITION PER SERVING

Calories 180 • Fat 2 g • Fiber 4 g • Protein 1 g • Carbohydrates 40 g

## steamed cabbage

MAKES 4 SERVINGS

This may not sound like much, but it is very cheap, it's healthy, and it tastes good.

**½ head green cabbage, shredded**
**Salt and freshly ground black pepper**

Fill a pot with ¼ inch of water and bring to a boil. Salt the water and add the cabbage; steam for about 10 minutes, or until tender. Drain, season with salt and pepper to taste, and serve hot.

NUTRITION PER SERVING

Calories 40 • Fat 0 g • Fiber 4 g • Protein 2 g • Carbohydrates 9 g

# simple green beans

MAKES 4 SERVINGS

Sometimes the best vegetables are the ones cooked simply so that their true flavors shine through. If you can, get organic green beans from a farmers' market, because they will be very fresh and delicately sweet.

**1 teaspoon extra-virgin olive oil**
**Salt (sea salt is best)**
**1 pound green beans, washed, ends trimmed off**
**3 tablespoons water**
**Parmesan cheese**
**Freshly ground black pepper (optional)**

1. Heat the olive oil in a large skillet over high heat. Add a pinch of salt to the pan, and then wait until the pan is very hot.
2. Toss the green beans into the pan; they should start sizzling and popping immediately. Sauté for 30 seconds, stirring constantly, then turn the heat down to medium. Add the water to the pan and cover with a large lid. Leave the beans to steam for several minutes until they are tender but still crisp.
3. Remove the beans from the pan and arrange them on a serving plate. Sprinkle with salt, Parmesan, and pepper, if using. Serve immediately.

NUTRITION PER SERVING

Calories 45 • Fat 1.5 g • Fiber 3 g • Protein 2 g • Carbohydrates 5 g

# glazed carrots

MAKES 4 SERVINGS

- ¼ cup water
- 4 medium carrots, peeled and chopped
- 1 tablespoon honey
- 1 teaspoon butter
- Nutmeg

1 Bring the water to a boil in a saucepan. Add the carrots, return to a boil, then reduce the heat and simmer, covered, until the carrots are tender, 7 to 10 minutes. Drain.

2 Add the honey and butter to the hot saucepan, and stir until they are melted together. Add the carrots and gently toss. Sprinkle with nutmeg to taste.

NUTRITION PER SERVING

Calories 50 • Fat 1 g • Fiber 2 g • Protein 1 g • Carbohydrates 10 g

# steamed asparagus

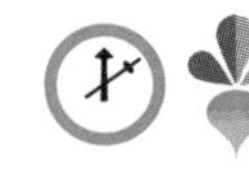

MAKES 4 SERVINGS

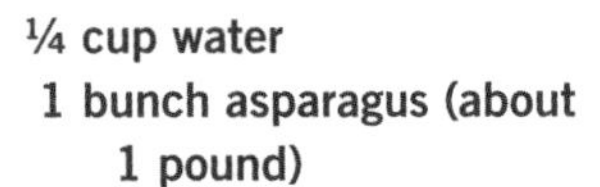

- ¼ cup water
- 1 bunch asparagus (about 1 pound)
- 1 tablespoon butter
- 1 teaspoon lemon juice

1 Bring the water to a boil in a large pot. Trim the ends from the asparagus, add them to the pot, cover, and cook until tender, 7 to 8 minutes.

2 Drain the asparagus and set on a serving dish. Sprinkle with slivers of butter and a spritz of lemon juice.

NUTRITION PER SERVING

Calories 45 • Fat 3.5 g • Fiber 2 g • Protein 2 g • Carbohydrates 3 g

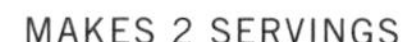

# grilled asparagus

MAKES 2 SERVINGS

**1 bunch asparagus (about 1 pound)**
**¼ cup extra-virgin olive oil**
**Salt (preferably sea salt)**

1. Preheat the grill.
2. Trim the ends from the asparagus, rinse the stalks, pat dry, and place in a baking dish. Drizzle the olive oil over the stalks, and sprinkle generously with salt. Use your hands to toss gently, making sure that all the stalks are coated.
3. Place the stalks directly on the grill rack over low heat. Grill until the stalks are very tender, 5 to 7 minutes, turning once.

**NOTE:** You can also make this recipe in a broiler or in an oven set at 450°F. Broil or roast the stalks in the baking dish until the stalks are very tender.

NUTRITION PER SERVING
Calories 300 • Fat 29 g • Fiber 3 g • Protein 5 g • Carbohydrates 6 g

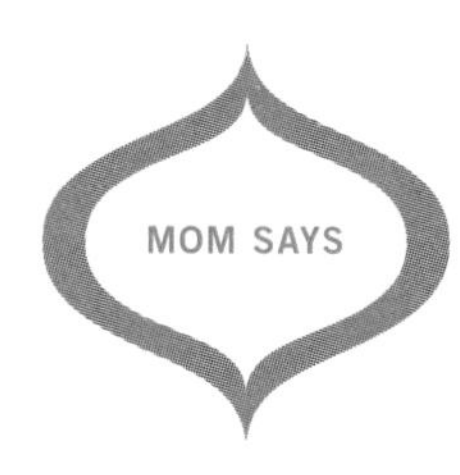


## lemon cubes

A splash of lemon juice will help to bring out the flavor of many fruits and vegetables, and it doesn't add a sour flavor. To keep fresh-squeezed lemon juice on hand, buy eight to ten lemons, squeeze their juice into an ice cube tray, and freeze. When the cubes are solid, empty them from the tray and put them in a ziplock freezer bag for safe storage in the freezer. Then, whenever you want to add lemon juice to steamed vegetables or other recipes, simply add a lemon cube.

# quick sautéed spinach

MAKES 2 SERVINGS

This recipe is fantastic and very fast. A whole pound of fresh spinach might look like a lot at first, but with a little heat it will shrink to a fraction of its original size. Turn this into a tasty main course by topping spinach with a grilled chicken breast or sautéed fish.

**1 tablespoon extra-virgin olive oil**
**1 tablespoon butter**
**1 pound fresh spinach, trimmed and washed**
**1 tablespoon lemon juice**
**¼ teaspoon ground nutmeg**
**Salt and freshly ground black pepper**

1. Heat the oil in a large skillet over medium heat for 2 minutes. Add the butter, letting it melt for a few seconds, and then add the spinach. If your skillet is not large enough to hold all of the raw spinach, add a handful, wait for it to cook down a little, then add the remaining leaves.
2. Cover the skillet and cook over medium heat for 3 to 4 minutes or until spinach is tender.
3. Remove the skillet from the heat, and add lemon juice and nutmeg. Give the spinach a good stir to combine the flavors. Season with salt and pepper to taste and serve warm.

NUTRITION PER SERVING
Calories 170 • Fat 14 g • Fiber 5 g • Protein 7 g • Carbohydrates 9 g

# roasted beets with onions

MAKES 2 SERVINGS

This is a great fall recipe that goes well with roast chicken. Leftovers can be puréed with chicken or vegetable broth, sprinkled with fresh dill, and served with sour cream for a great soup.

**1½ pounds beets (golden beets are particularly good, but any color will do)**
**1 large sweet onion**
**1 tablespoon extra-virgin olive oil**
**2 teaspoons dried rosemary**
**¼ teaspoon salt (sea salt works best)**
**Freshly ground black pepper**

1. Preheat the oven to 425°F.
2. Wash, peel, and chop the beets into ½-inch chunks. Peel the onion and chop into ½-inch chunks.
3. Toss together all of the ingredients (it's okay if the onion separates into slices) and place in a roasting pan. Cover with aluminum foil and roast until tender, 45 to 60 minutes.

NUTRITION PER SERVING

Calories 220 • Fat 8 g • Fiber 8 g • Protein 4 g • Carbohydrates 37 g

# grilled eggplant

MAKES 4 SERVINGS

A simple preparation for eggplant, this side dish is great when you're grilling other foods for supper.

**1 medium eggplant**
**Vegetable marinade (see our recipe on page 250)**

1. Peel the eggplant, then slice into ½-inch rounds. Soak in the marinade for 1 hour.
2. Preheat the broiler.
3. Place the slices on a rack set on a baking sheet and broil until hot and soft, about 5 minutes per side.

NUTRITION PER SERVING

Calories 170 • Fat 14 g • Fiber 4 g • Protein 1 g • Carbohydrates 10 g

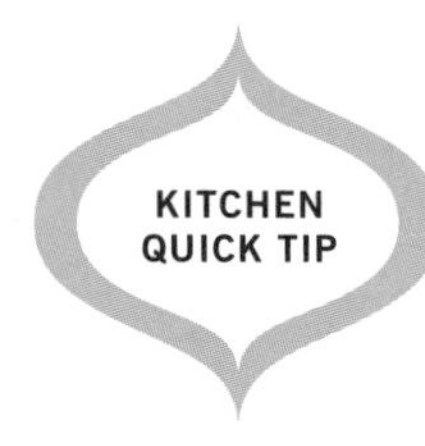


## the truth about eggplant

Did you know that eggplant is technically not a vegetable but a berry? Also, eggplant is an excellent source of potassium.

# sweet winter squash

MAKES 4 SERVINGS

This is a great fall dish. The recipe works with a variety of squashes — we recommend acorn or butternut.

**2 small acorn squash or 1 large butternut squash (about 1 pound total)**
**2 teaspoons butter**
**4 teaspoons packed brown sugar**

1. Preheat the oven to 350°F.
2. Cut the squash in half. (If you're using 1 large squash, cut it into quarters.) Scoop out the seeds.
3. With a fork, poke holes in the flesh of the squash. Drop ½ teaspoon of butter and 1 teaspoon of sugar into the center of each piece.
4. Place the squash face up in a baking pan. Cover with aluminum foil and bake until soft, about 40 minutes.

NUTRITION PER SERVING
Calories 120 • Fat 2 g • Fiber 3 g • Protein 2 g • Carbohydrates 27 g

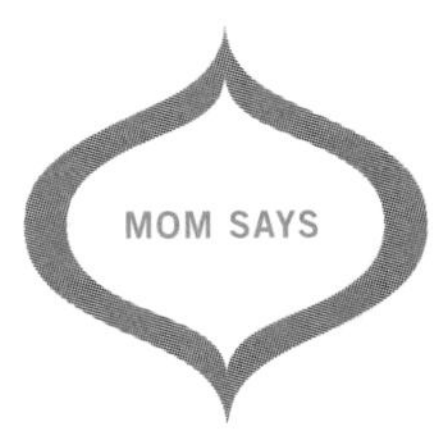


## quick cooking

To reduce the cooking time for this recipe, you can place the cut pieces of squash in a microwave-safe dish and microwave on high for 8 minutes before baking. This will reduce the oven baking time to about 15 minutes.

# balsamic tomatoes

MAKES 4 SERVINGS

**2 medium tomatoes, cut into thick slices**
**½ medium onion, finely chopped**
**3 tablespoons balsamic vinegar**
**2 teaspoons extra-virgin olive oil**
**Freshly ground black pepper**

1. Arrange the tomato slices on a plate and sprinkle with the onion.
2. Drizzle the vinegar and oil over the tomatoes, and season with pepper to taste. Marinate for at least 5 minutes before serving.

NUTRITION PER SERVING
Calories 260 • Fat 2.5 g • Fiber 1 g • Protein 1 g • Carbohydrates 7 g

# sweet potato fries

MAKES 4 SERVINGS

**2 large sweet potatoes**
**2 tablespoons extra-virgin olive oil**
**2 teaspoons hot sauce**
**Salt and freshly ground black pepper**

1. Preheat the oven to 500°F.
2. Scrub the sweet potatoes and cut them into wedges about ¾ inch wide. Combine the olive oil, hot sauce, and salt and pepper to taste in a large bowl. Add the sweet potato wedges and toss to coat evenly.
3. Set the potato wedges in a single layer on a baking sheet and bake for 20 to 30 minutes, until nicely browned, flipping them once.

NUTRITION PER SERVING
Calories 90 • Fat 3.5 g • Fiber 2 g • Protein 1 g • Carbohydrates 14 g

# broccoli with onions and soy sauce

MAKES 4 SERVINGS

This recipe is great served over rice for a quick vegetarian meal.

**4 cups broccoli florets**
**1 teaspoon sesame oil**
**1 onion, chopped**
**⅓ cup low-sodium soy sauce**

1. Place the broccoli in a large pot and add ¼ to ½ inch of water. Bring to a boil, reduce the heat, and steam, covered, for 5 to 7 minutes, until bright green and crisp (you don't want it to be fully cooked).
2. Heat the oil in a large pan over medium heat. Add the onion and sauté until it's just translucent. Add the broccoli and soy sauce and cook, stirring often, for 5 minutes, or until the broccoli is tender.

NUTRITION PER SERVING
Calories 60 • Fat 1.5 g • Fiber 3 g • Protein 4 g • Carbohydrates 8 g

# vegetable and herb rice pilaf

MAKES 4 SERVINGS

This quick recipe is hearty enough to serve as a main dish.

- **1 cup broccoli florets**
- **2 tablespoons extra-virgin olive oil**
- **2 garlic cloves, finely chopped**
- **1 small onion, chopped**
- **½ cup canned kidney beans, rinsed and drained**
- **½ cup diced tomatoes**
- **½ teaspoon dried basil**
- **½ teaspoon dried oregano**
- **Salt and freshly ground black pepper**
- **½ cup vegetable broth**
- **1 cup cooked rice**

1. Put an inch of water into a pot. Add the broccoli. Bring to a boil, reduce heat, cover, and steam until the broccoli is tender, about 7 minutes.
2. While the broccoli is cooking, heat the olive oil in a large skillet over medium heat. Add the garlic and onion and sauté until the onion is translucent.
3. Add the kidney beans, tomatoes, basil, oregano, and salt and pepper to taste to the skillet. Reduce the heat to medium-low, cover, and continue to cook, stirring occasionally.
4. Add the cooked broccoli, vegetable broth, and rice to the skillet. Bring to a boil, reduce heat, and simmer, covered, for 5 minutes, stirring occasionally. Serve hot.

**NOTE:** This recipe leaves you with leftover kidney beans. Store them in an airtight container in the refrigerator and toss a handful in soups or salads.

NUTRITION PER SERVING

Calories 210 • Fat 7 g • Fiber 4 g • Protein 5 g • Carbohydrates 31 g

# island teriyaki marinade

MAKES 4 SERVINGS

You can use this marinade for meats, fish, vegetables, and just about anything else you can think of. Depending on the thickness of the food, you'll want to marinate for at least 1 or 2 hours before cooking.

- **½ cup low-sodium soy sauce**
- **¼ cup packed brown sugar**
- **1½ tablespoons extra-virgin olive oil**
- **1 tablespoon freshly grated ginger**
- **¼ teaspoon freshly ground black pepper**
- **2 garlic cloves, minced**

Combine all ingredients and mix well.

NUTRITION PER SERVING

Calories 130 • Fat 5 g • Fiber 0 g • Protein 2 g • Carbohydrates 17 g

## 6 quick recipes for rice

- Add dehydrated chicken soup mix (use a low-sodium variety, if available) to the boiling water, and mix in some cooked chicken before serving.
- Add onion soup mix (use a low-sodium variety, if available) to the boiling water, and mix in sautéed mushrooms before serving.
- Cook the rice in vegetable broth (use a low-sodium variety, if available), and mix in steamed or grilled vegetables before serving.
- Mix salsa in with the cooked rice, and top with a sprinkle of cheese.
- Stir curry powder and cooked chicken in with the cooked rice.
- For quick red beans and rice, heat up some canned red beans. Stir in onions, celery, green pepper, garlic, and oregano to taste. Serve over white rice.

## vegetable marinade

MAKES 4 SERVINGS

Use this marinade for vegetables such as zucchini, eggplant, cucumber, and mushrooms.

**¼ cup extra-virgin olive oil**
**¼ cup balsamic vinegar**
**1 tablespoon water**
**1 garlic clove, minced**
**1 teaspoon dried oregano**
**½ teaspoon freshly ground black pepper**
**½ teaspoon salt**

Combine all ingredients and mix well.

NUTRITION PER SERVING

Calories 140 • Fat 14 g • Fiber 0 g • Protein 0 g • Carbohydrates 3 g

## soy-peanut sauce

MAKES 4 SERVINGS

Use this sauce over rice and vegetables or as a marinade for chicken or beef. The measurements given here are just a guideline; the proportions are extremely flexible and can be changed to suit your taste or the ingredients you have on hand.

**½ cup low-sodium soy sauce**
**½ cup honey**
**2 tablespoons peanut butter**
**2 tablespoons freshly grated ginger**
**1 tablespoon lime juice**
**2 garlic cloves, minced**

Whisk together all ingredients in a small bowl.

NUTRITION PER SERVING

Calories 210 • Fat 4 g • Fiber 1 g • Protein 5 g • Carbohydrates 40 g

## mom's bbq sauce

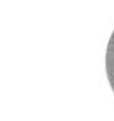

MAKES 10 SERVINGS

- **½ tablespoon extra-virgin olive oil**
- **1 small yellow onion, finely chopped**
- **⅔ cup ketchup**
- **2 tablespoons lemon juice**
- **2 tablespoons red wine vinegar**
- **1 tablespoon mustard**
- **1 tablespoon Worcestershire sauce**
- **1 teaspoon hot sauce**
- **½ teaspoon freshly ground black pepper**
- **Pinch of salt**

Heat the oil in a saucepan over medium heat. Add the onion and sauté until translucent, about 5 minutes. Add the remaining ingredients; stir well. Simmer for 15 minutes, stirring occasionally.

NUTRITION PER SERVING

Calories 30 • Fat 1 g • Fiber 0 g • Protein 1 g • Carbohydrates 6 g

## apple cinnamon purée

MAKES 6 SERVINGS

Serve over plain fruit salads or as a summer dip for sliced fruit.

- **1 medium apple, peeled, cored, and chopped**
- **⅓ cup skim milk**
- **⅔ cup nonfat plain yogurt**
- **2 teaspoons sugar**
- **2 teaspoons cinnamon**

Combine all of the ingredients in a blender or food processor, and blend until smooth.

NUTRITION PER SERVING

Calories 40 • Fat 0 g • Fiber 1 g • Protein 2 g • Carbohydrates 9 g

# chicken gravy

MAKES 8 SERVINGS

This also works well for beef — just switch the broth.

**2 tablespoons all-purpose flour**
**1 cup low-sodium chicken broth**

In a saucepan, slowly whisk the flour into the broth until it reaches an even consistency. Bring the broth to a boil, reduce heat, and simmer, stirring often, until the sauce thickens.

NUTRITION PER SERVING
Calories 10 • Fat 0 g • Fiber 0 g • Protein 1 g • Carbohydrates 2 g

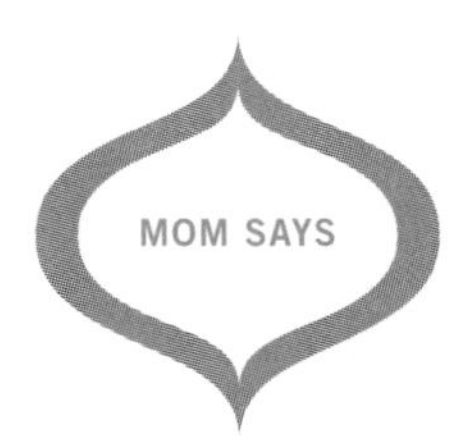


## gravy tips

- If you need to thicken a gravy or cream sauce, try adding a little flour or cornstarch. Stir it into the sauce until it has been absorbed.
- The flour or cornstarch in your gravy should be mixed with cold liquid — either will form lumps when mixed with hot liquid. If the gravy or sauce is already hot, mix the flour with a bit of cold water before adding it.
- If you overspice a gravy, add a peeled raw potato to absorb some of the seasoning. Let it soak in the gravy for a while, and then remove and discard it.

# mango salsa

MAKES 4 SERVINGS

A tropical alternative to the traditional red and green salsas.

1 mango, pitted, peeled, and chopped
½ jalapeño, seeded, deveined, and diced
¼ red onion, chopped
Several sprigs of fresh cilantro, chopped
1 tablespoon lime juice

Combine all ingredients. Let sit for at least 10 minutes before serving to allow the flavors to blend.

NUTRITION PER SERVING
Calories 40 • Fat 0 g • Fiber 1 g • Protein 0 g • Carbohydrates 10 g

# cocktail sauce

MAKES 8 SERVINGS

Most commonly used as a dip for chilled shrimp.

½ cup ketchup
2 tablespoons horseradish
2 tablespoons lemon juice

Combine all ingredients and stir well. Serve chilled.

NUTRITION PER SERVING
Calories 15 • Fat 0 g • Fiber 0 g • Protein 0 g • Carbohydrates 4 g

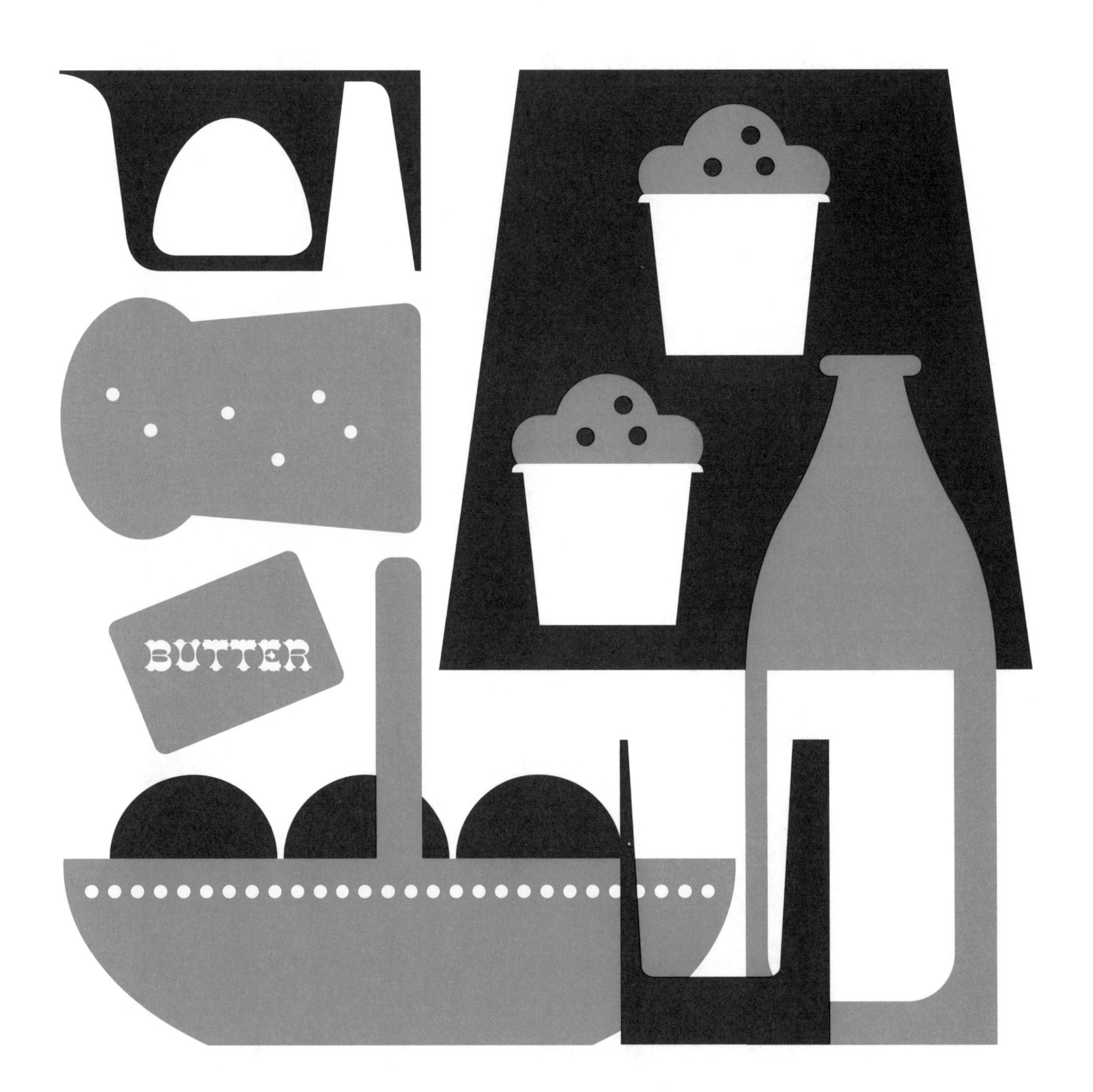
BUTTER

# chapter 11

## breads, biscuits & muffins

Everybody loves biting into a warm slice of bread fresh from the oven. However, when brainstorming on what type of recipes to include in this book, we originally left out breads. Why? Because of the time commitment involved. Well, a little more research helped us to discover that breads can be as simple and quick to make as anything else. We've found some recipes that take very little time to prepare — no long hours of kneading — and leave the hard and lengthy work to the oven. Once the aroma begins to fill your apartment and escape out the door, you may find friends suddenly appearing on your doorstep. So enjoy your bread in good company.

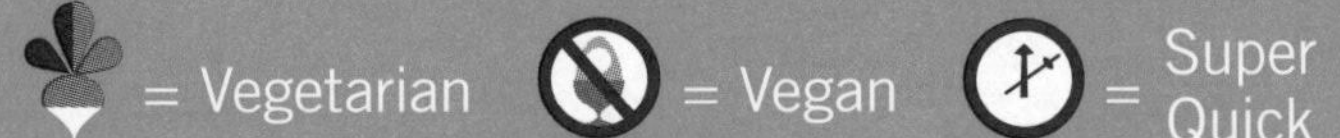
= Vegetarian
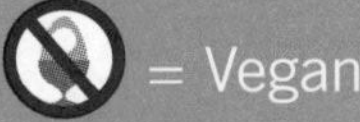
= Vegan
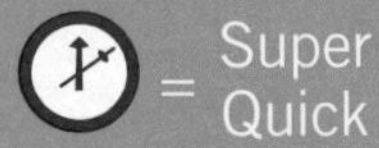
= Super Quick
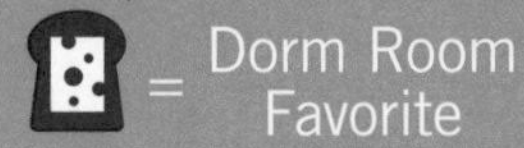
= Dorm Room Favorite

# whole-wheat honey biscuits

MAKES 12 BISCUITS

These biscuits are great with jam for a quick breakfast. The mixing and the baking won't take long, but you do have to wait for the dough to rise (30 to 40 minutes), so save this recipe for a day when you'll be studying at home.

**1 cup lukewarm water**
**2 tablespoons active dry yeast**
**2½ cups whole-wheat flour**
**5 teaspoons honey**
**Cooking spray**

1. Pour the water into a large mixing bowl. Stir in the yeast and let sit until the mixture is slightly bubbly, about 10 minutes. Add the flour and honey; mix well.
2. Lightly coat a 12-cup muffin tin with cooking spray. Fill each cup halfway with batter.
3. Let the muffin tin sit somewhere warm (next to a warm radiator, on top of a running dryer, or next to a preheating oven) until the batter has doubled in size, 30 to 40 minutes.
4. Near the end of the rising time, preheat the oven to 350°F.
5. Bake for 20 minutes. Let the biscuits sit for 5 to 10 minutes before removing from their tins.

NUTRITION PER SERVING

Calories 100 • Fat 0.5 g • Fiber 3 g • Protein 4 g • Carbohydrates 21 g

# pumpkin bread

MAKES 10 SERVINGS

Pumpkin is very good for you, and the canned stuff is just as good as fresh.

- **Cooking spray**
- **2 eggs, beaten**
- **1 cup sugar**
- **¼ cup vegetable oil**
- **¼ cup applesauce (see page 235 for our recipe)**
- **1 (10-ounce) can pumpkin pie filling**
- **1½ cups all-purpose flour**
- **1 teaspoon baking powder**
- **1 teaspoon baking soda**
- **1½ teaspoons cinnamon**
- **½ teaspoon salt**

1. Preheat the oven to 375°F. Lightly grease a 9- by 5-inch loaf pan with cooking spray.
2. Combine the eggs and sugar in a medium bowl. Mix in the oil and applesauce. Add the pumpkin pie filling and mix thoroughly.
3. Stir together the flour, baking powder, baking soda, cinnamon, and salt in a separate bowl. Add the dry ingredients to the pumpkin mixture and mix thoroughly.
4. Pour the batter into the prepared loaf pan. Bake for 1 hour, until a knife inserted into the middle of the loaf comes out clean.

NUTRITION PER SERVING

Calories 240 • Fat 7 g • Fiber 3 g • Protein 3 g • Carbohydrates 43 g

# blueberry scones

MAKES 6 SCONES

For a different taste, substitute an equal amount of other berries or fruits for the blueberries.

- **Cooking spray**
- **1 cup all-purpose flour**
- **3 tablespoons sugar**
- **1½ teaspoons baking powder**
- **½ teaspoon salt**
- **1 teaspoon lemon zest**
- **2 tablespoons cold butter, cut into pea-size pieces**
- **1 egg**
- **3 tablespoons skim milk**
- **½ cup blueberries**

1. Preheat the oven to 400°F. Coat a baking sheet with cooking spray.
2. Combine the flour, sugar, baking powder, salt, and zest in a mixing bowl. Add the butter and blend with a fork until the mixture forms rough crumbs.
3. Beat together the egg and milk in a separate bowl. Add the liquid to the dry ingredients and mix thoroughly. Gently fold in the blueberries and stir well, until the dough comes cleanly off the sides of bowl.
4. Flour a large, flat work surface. Knead the dough on the floured surface until it sticks together well. Sprinkle in more flour if it's too sticky and clings to your hands.
5. Form the dough into 6 balls. Place them on the prepared baking sheet, and flatten each to about ½-inch thickness.
6. Bake for about 12 minutes, until light brown on top. Cool before serving.

NUTRITION PER SERVING

Calories 160 • Fat 5 g • Fiber 1 g • Protein 4 g • Carbohydrates 25 g

# zucchini bread

MAKES 12 SERVINGS

This quick bread is a great use for extra garden zucchini you might pick up at a farmers' market.

- **Cooking spray**
- **1½ cups grated zucchini**
- **1 cup all-purpose flour**
- **½ cup rolled oats**
- **2 teaspoons cinnamon**
- **1½ teaspoons baking powder**
- **¼ teaspoon freshly grated ginger (optional)**
- **1 cup packed brown sugar**
- **⅓ cup vegetable oil**
- **⅓ cup applesauce (see page 235 for our recipe)**
- **2 eggs, beaten**
- **2 teaspoons vanilla extract**
- **½ teaspoon salt**

1. Preheat the oven to 350°F. Lightly grease a 9- by 5-inch loaf pan with cooking spray.
2. Combine the zucchini, flour, oats, cinnamon, baking powder, and ginger, if using, in a large bowl. Mix well. Blend in the sugar, oil, applesauce, eggs, vanilla, and salt. Stir until the batter is smooth.
3. Pour the batter into the prepared loaf pan and bake for 45 minutes, or until a knife inserted into the center comes out clean. Cool the loaf on a rack before removing it from the pan.

NUTRITION PER SERVING

Calories 200 • Fat 7 g • Fiber 1 g • Protein 3 g • Carbohydrates 30 g

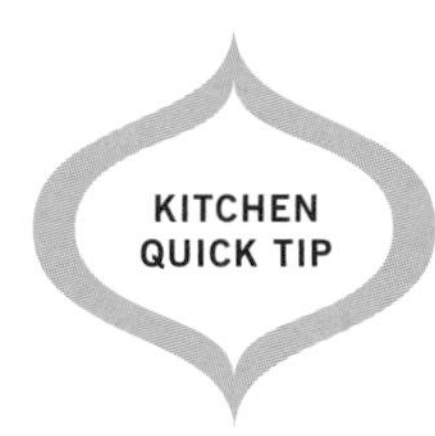


## adding fiber

Include extra fiber in your breads, muffins, and cookies by adding a touch of wheat bran or oat bran, some nuts, or dried fruit such as raisins, apricots, or dates.

# beer bread

MAKES 8 SERVINGS

This is a speedy bread recipe; it's best served with jam or honey.

**3 cups all-purpose flour**
**3 tablespoons sugar**
**4 tablespoons active dry yeast**
**1 (12-ounce) bottle beer**
**Cooking spray**

1. Stir together the flour, sugar, and yeast in a large bowl. Add the beer and mix well.
2. Spray a loaf pan with cooking spray; pour in the batter. Place in a cold oven and set to 350°F. Bake for 40 to 45 minutes, until a knife inserted in the center comes out clean. Cool the loaf on a rack before removing it from the pan.

NUTRITION PER SERVING
Calories 230 • Fat 0.5 g • Fiber 3 g • Protein 7 g • Carbohydrates 44 g

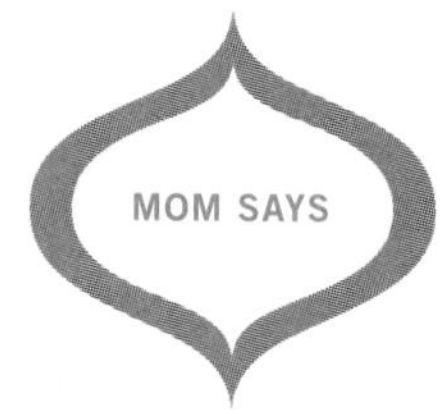


## to spray or not?

Cooking spray is great to have in your kitchen, but you can always use a bit of butter to grease your baking pans. The butter that's left on the wrapper after you unwrap a stick is usually plenty.

# southwestern corn bread

MAKES 6 SERVINGS

Corn bread is a delicious accompaniment to southwestern dishes, soups, and salads.

**Cooking spray**
**1 (10-ounce) package corn bread mix, plus any ingredients called for in the package directions**
**1 (7-ounce) can creamed corn**
**1 tablespoon chopped jalapeño pepper**
**Honey**

1. Preheat the oven to 375°F. Lightly grease a 9- by 5-inch loaf pan with cooking spray.
2. Prepare the corn bread batter according to the package directions. Stir in the creamed corn and chopped jalapeño.
3. Pour the batter into the prepared loaf pan. Bake for 20 minutes, or until the top of the loaf springs back when touched in the center.
4. Spread honey over the top immediately upon removing the pan from the oven. Let stand for at least 5 minutes before serving.

NUTRITION PER SERVING

Calories 220 • Fat 2.5 g • Fiber 3 g • Protein 8 g • Carbohydrates 44 g

# bran muffins

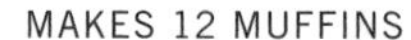

MAKES 12 MUFFINS

The applesauce and milk keep the bran cereal from tasting too dry.

**Cooking spray**
**1 cup all-purpose flour**
**¾ cup bran cereal (flakes)**
**⅔ cup sugar**
**2 teaspoons baking soda**
**1 teaspoon baking powder**
**½ teaspoon cinnamon**
**¼ teaspoon salt**
**1 egg**
**½ cup skim milk**
**⅓ cup applesauce (see page 235 for our recipe)**
**½ cup orange juice**

1. Preheat the oven to 350°F. Lightly grease a 12-cup muffin tin with cooking spray.
2. Combine the flour, cereal, sugar, baking soda, baking powder, cinnamon, and salt in a large bowl. Mix gently (don't crush the bran flakes).
3. Beat the egg in a separate bowl. Add the milk and applesauce, and mix until smooth. Combine the egg mixture with the dry ingredients and add the orange juice. Mix gently.
4. Fill the prepared muffin cups about ¾ full with the batter. Bake for about 15 minutes, until a knife inserted in the center comes out clean.

NUTRITION PER SERVING

Calories 110 • Fat 0.5 g • Fiber 1 g • Protein 2 g • Carbohydrates 25 g

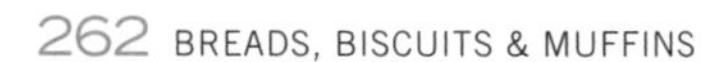

# blueberry muffins with oats

MAKES 15 MUFFINS

- Cooking spray
- 1½ cups all-purpose flour
- 1 cup old-fashioned rolled oats
- ½ cup sugar
- 4 teaspoons baking powder
- ½ teaspoon salt
- ½ teaspoon nutmeg
- 1 cup skim milk
- 1 egg
- 1 teaspoon vanilla extract
- 3 tablespoons applesauce (see page 235 for our recipe)
- 1½ cups blueberries

1. Preheat the oven to 350°F. Lightly grease a 12-cup muffin tin with cooking spray.
2. Combine the flour, oats, sugar, baking powder, salt, and nutmeg in a large bowl.
3. Mix together the milk, egg, and vanilla in a separate bowl. Stir in the applesauce.
4. Combine the wet ingredients with the dry ingredients and mix thoroughly. Gently fold in the blueberries.
5. Fill the prepared muffin cups about ¾ full with the batter. Bake for 15 to 20 minutes, until a knife inserted in the center comes out clean.

NUTRITION PER SERVING

Calories 110 • Fat 1 g • Fiber 1 g • Protein 3 g • Carbohydrates 23 g

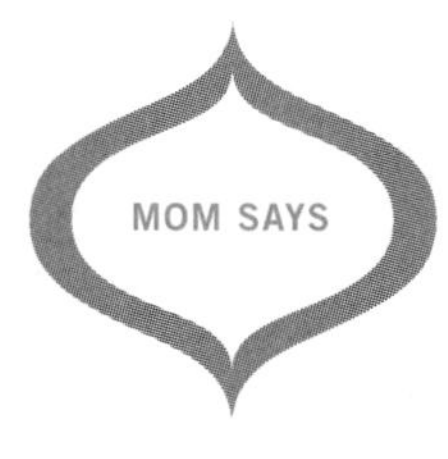


## keeping milk on hand

Keep a bag of nonfat dry milk powder in your cupboard to use in making breads. This will save you money in the long run, especially if you're not a milk drinker, since you won't have to buy carton upon carton of fresh milk for every recipe you try. When used in breads and muffins, rehydrated nonfat dry milk tastes the same as the fresh stuff.

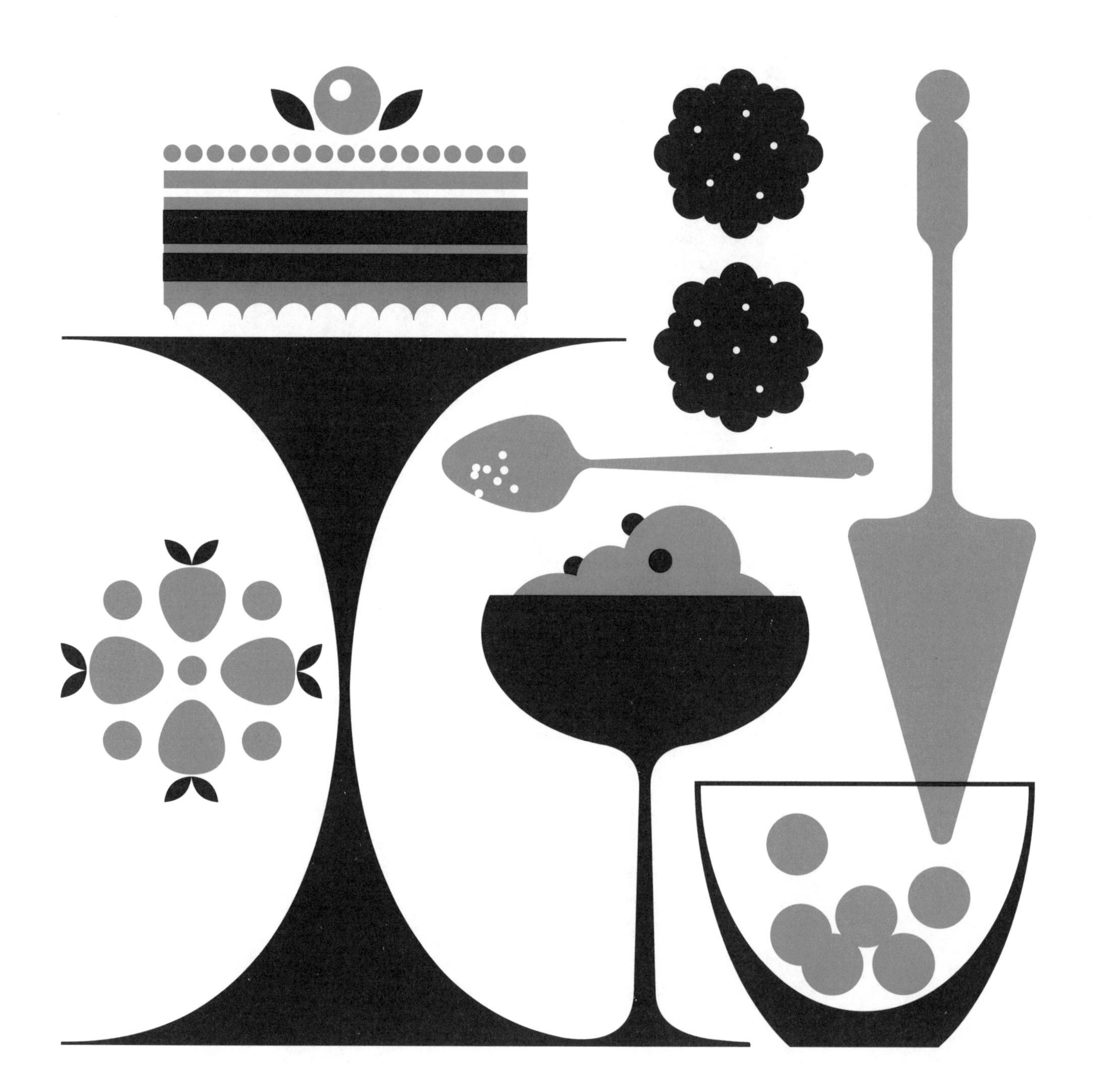

# chapter 12

## desserts

We had trouble keeping this section short. Always an anticipated course during a meal, dessert lies close to practically everyone's heart. We've tried our best to provide you with a few recipes that make our favorite part of the meal just a little healthier — but for all those who crave the traditional moist, rich flavor of a delicious chocolate cake fresh from the oven, we've included one of those as well.

Some hints in this section and throughout the book provide you with options for making a recipe healthier while at the same time maintaining the recipe's texture and flavor. Don't go overboard, though — this is still dessert, and it wouldn't be dessert if it didn't include the temptation for just one more bite, offset by the growing pressure of your belt buckle. Have fun here, and when done, sit back and relax. If you've made it through cooking an entire meal on your own, then smile, feel accomplished, and pick up your fork for another bite of dessert.

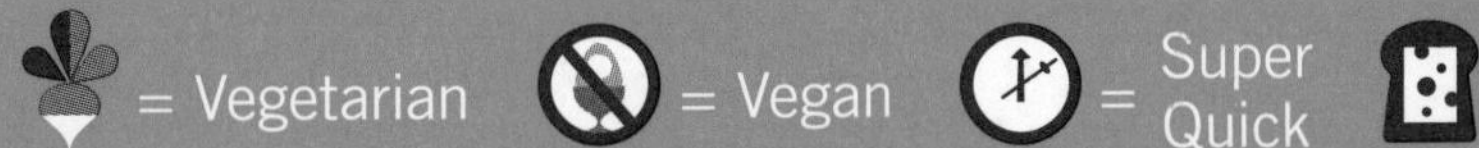
= Vegetarian
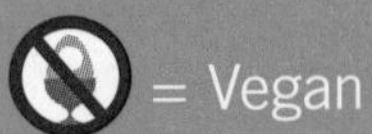
= Vegan
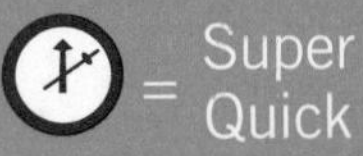
= Super Quick
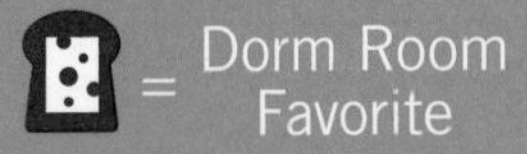
= Dorm Room Favorite

# carrot cake

MAKES 12 SERVINGS

This cake is so rich and moist you won't miss the cream cheese frosting usually added to carrot cake.

**Cooking spray**
**1⅓ cups all-purpose flour**
**1 cup sugar**
**1½ teaspoons baking soda**
**1 teaspoon baking powder**
**1 teaspoon cinnamon**
**½ teaspoon nutmeg**
**Pinch of salt**
**⅓ cup vegetable oil**
**⅓ cup applesauce (see page 235 for our recipe)**
**2 eggs, beaten**
**1½ cups grated carrots**

1. Preheat the oven to 350°F. Lightly grease and flour a 9- by 5-inch loaf pan with cooking spray.
2. Stir together the flour, sugar, baking soda, baking powder, cinnamon, and nutmeg in a large bowl. Sprinkle in a pinch of salt.
3. Stir in the oil, applesauce, and eggs. Add the carrots and mix well.
4. Pour the batter into the prepared loaf pan and bake for about 30 minutes, or until a knife inserted into the cake's center comes out dry. Cool on a rack before removing from the pan.

NUTRITION PER SERVING

Calories 180 • Fat 7 g • Fiber 1 g • Protein 2 g • Carbohydrates 28 g

# spice loaf

MAKES 10 SERVINGS

Spice loaf is great anytime: for breakfast, a snack, or dessert. While it is convenient to have an electric mixer of some sort when making this recipe, it's not essential.

- **Cooking spray**
- **1½ cups all-purpose flour**
- **½ cup sugar**
- **1½ teaspoons baking powder**
- **1 teaspoon cinnamon**
- **½ teaspoon salt**
- **½ teaspoon nutmeg**
- **5 tablespoons cold butter, cut into pea-size pieces**
- **2 egg whites**
- **⅔ cup skim milk**

1. Preheat the oven to 350°F. Lightly grease a 9- by 5-inch loaf pan with cooking spray.
2. Combine the flour, sugar, baking powder, cinnamon, salt, and nutmeg in a large mixing bowl. Mix well. Add the butter and mix thoroughly. Stir in the egg whites and milk.
3. Pour the batter into the prepared loaf pan. Place the pan on a baking sheet in the center of the oven. Bake for 45 minutes, or until the top is golden brown. Cool the loaf on a rack before removing it from the pan.

NUTRITION PER SERVING

Calories 170 • Fat 6 g • Fiber 1 g • Protein 3 g • Carbohydrates 26 g

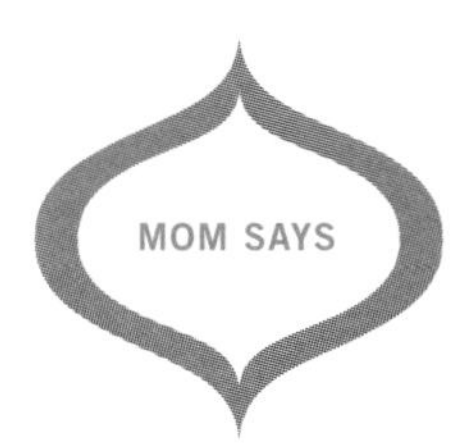


## cut out the fat

If you add too much cooking spray to your baking pan, just wipe out the excess with a paper towel.

# banana chocolate chip muffins

MAKES 12 MUFFINS

Bananas and chocolate are always a winning combination.

- Cooking spray
- 1 cup sugar
- ½ cup vegetable shortening (preferably nonhydrogenated)
- 2 cups all-purpose flour
- 2 eggs
- 3 large (or 5 small) very ripe bananas
- 1 teaspoon baking soda
- 1 teaspoon baking powder
- ½ teaspoon salt
- ⅔ cup mini chocolate chips

1. Preheat the oven to 350°F. Grease a 12-cup muffin tin with cooking spray.
2. Cream together the sugar and shortening in a mixing bowl. Add 1 tablespoon of the flour to the mixture. Beat in the eggs 1 at a time.
3. Mash the bananas to a soft pulp in a separate bowl.
4. Set aside ½ cup of the flour. Add the remaining flour and the banana pulp to the creamed mixture, mixing it in bit by bit.
5. Stir together the reserved ½ cup of flour with the baking soda, baking powder, and salt. Add the chocolate chips, tossing to coat.
6. Combine the dry and creamed mixtures; stir well. Pour the batter into the prepared muffin tins and bake for 25 minutes, or until a knife inserted in the center of a muffin comes out clean.

NUTRITION PER SERVING

Calories 320 • Fat 13 g • Fiber 1 g • Protein 4 g • Carbohydrates 49 g

## peaches and cream

  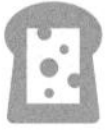

MAKES 4 SERVINGS

4 whole peaches, peeled, pitted, and chopped
Juice of 1 lemon
½ cup low-fat whipped cream
¼ cup packed brown sugar

1. Preheat the broiler.
2. Arrange the peaches in a baking dish, spreading them out evenly, and squeeze lemon juice over the top. Cover evenly with whipped cream, then sprinkle with sugar. Broil for 4 minutes, or until the top begins to turn golden.

NUTRITION PER SERVING

Calories 140 • Fat 2.5 g • Fiber 2 g • Protein 1 g • Carbohydrates 31 g

## tropical fruit salad

  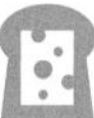

MAKES 4 SERVINGS

1 mango, peeled, pitted, and sliced
2 bananas, peeled and sliced
2 kiwi, peeled and sliced
3 tablespoons orange juice
1 tablespoon lemon juice

Mix together the mango, bananas, and kiwi. Stir in the orange and lemon juices.

NUTRITION PER SERVING

Calories 110 • Fat 0.5 g • Fiber 4 g • Protein 1 g • Carbohydrates 29 g

# apple cobbler

MAKES 6 SERVINGS

This easy dessert can also be made with pears, peaches, or any other fruit that you desire.

**4 large apples (McIntosh are best), peeled and thinly sliced**
**4 tablespoons all-purpose flour**
**3 tablespoons apple juice**
**1 teaspoon cinnamon**
**Pinch of nutmeg**
**7 tablespoons graham cracker crumbs**
**1 tablespoon butter, melted**
**1 tablespoon water**

1. Preheat the oven to 375°F.
2. Toss together the apples, 2 tablespoons of the flour, and the apple juice in a loaf pan, until the apple slices are well coated.
3. Combine the remaining 2 tablespoons of flour, cinnamon, nutmeg, and graham cracker crumbs in a separate bowl. Stir in the butter and water. Mix until pea-size clumps form.
4. Spread the graham cracker topping over the apples. Bake for 30 minutes, or until the topping is lightly browned.

NUTRITION PER SERVING

Calories 130 • Fat 3 g • Fiber 3 g • Protein 1 g • Carbohydrates 27 g

# granny's apple pie fruit salad

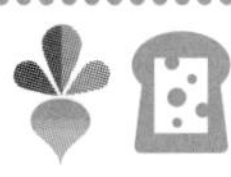

MAKES 2 SERVINGS

Nothing says home like apple pie! Each helping of this dish contains two servings of fruit, and it's loaded with good protein and carbohydrates to keep your mind sharp.

- **⅓ cup water**
- **⅓ cup lemon juice**
- **2 apples, cored and chopped (one each of Golden Delicious and Red Delicious is pretty and tasty)**
- **1 cup nonfat vanilla yogurt**
- **¼ cup dried cranberries**
- **¼ cup raisins**
- **¼ cup chopped pecans**
- **1 teaspoon cinnamon**
- **½ teaspoon ground cloves**
- **½ teaspoon nutmeg**
- **1 cup cinnamon granola**

1. Combine the water and lemon juice in a medium bowl. Add the apples, toss to coat, and let sit for 10 minutes. (This will prevent the apples from turning brown.)
2. In a separate bowl, combine the yogurt, cranberries, raisins, pecans, and spices. Drain the apples, pat dry, and stir them into the yogurt mixture. Divide the mixture into 2 serving bowls, and top each with half of the granola. Enjoy immediately or cover, refrigerate, and savor later.

NUTRITION PER SERVING

Calories 350 • Fat 8 g • Fiber 7 g • Protein 9 g • Carbohydrates 60 g

# strawberry shortcake

MAKES 10 SERVINGS

This recipe makes about ten biscuits. If you're not planning to eat ten strawberry shortcakes, you may want to halve the ingredients for the strawberry topping, but we recommend that you go ahead and make the full ten biscuits anyway. They are great plain or spread with jam for breakfast or a quick snack.

**½ cup skim milk**
**1 tablespoon lemon juice**
**1¼ cups all-purpose flour**
**6 tablespoons sugar**
**½ teaspoon baking powder**
**2 tablespoons chilled butter, cut into 8 pieces**
**2 tablespoons light cream or half-and-half**
**2 cups sliced strawberries**
**Light whipped cream to taste (about 1 tablespoon per person)**

1. Preheat the oven to 475°F.
2. Stir together the milk and lemon juice in a small bowl.
3. Mix together the flour, sugar, and baking powder in a separate large bowl. Add the butter and cream until the mixture is of an even consistency. Add the milk mixture and combine thoroughly.
4. Drop the batter in spoonfuls onto an ungreased baking sheet. Bake for about 15 minutes, until the biscuits are golden brown.
5. Serve the biscuits covered with strawberries and topped with whipped cream.

NUTRITION PER SERVING

Calories 140 • Fat 4 g • Fiber 1 g • Protein 22 g • Carbohydrates 24 g

# fruit cobbler

MAKES 8 SERVINGS

The crumbly, golden brown cake topping is just enough to hold together all the fruit and nuts.

- **1 (21-ounce) can cherry pie filling**
- **1 (14-ounce) can crushed pineapple, undrained**
- **1 (18.25-ounce) box yellow cake mix**
- **1 cup (2 sticks) butter, melted**
- **⅔ cup coconut**
- **⅔ cup chopped nuts, such as pecans or walnuts**
- **Ice cream or whipped cream for serving**

1. Preheat the oven to 350°F.
2. Spread the pie filling and pineapple in the bottom of a 9- by 13-inch baking pan. Sprinkle with the dry cake mix and drizzle with melted butter. Sprinkle with the coconut and chopped nuts.
3. Bake for about 1 hour, until the topping is golden brown and set. Watch closely during the final 15 minutes. If the topping becomes too browned, cover lightly with aluminum foil.
4. Serve warm or cold with ice cream or whipped cream. (Canned whipped cream works well on picnics.)

NUTRITION PER SERVING

Calories 710 • Fat 42 g • Fiber 4 g • Protein 5 g • Carbohydrates 83 g

# apple custard

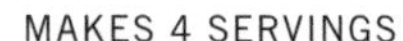

MAKES 4 SERVINGS

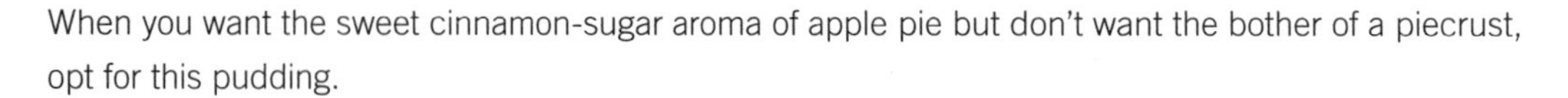

When you want the sweet cinnamon-sugar aroma of apple pie but don't want the bother of a piecrust, opt for this pudding.

**1 tablespoon butter**
**3 cups peeled and sliced apples**
**¼ cup skim milk**
**3 tablespoons all-purpose flour**
**1½ tablespoons sugar**
**1 egg, beaten**
**1½ tablespoons baking powder**
**1 teaspoon cinnamon**

1. Preheat the oven to 350°F.
2. Melt the butter in a skillet over medium heat. Add the apples and sauté until tender.
3. Combine the milk, flour, sugar, egg, baking powder, and cinnamon in a mixing bowl and blend until smooth.
4. Spread the apples in a shallow baking dish, forming a level layer. Pour in the batter, covering the apples completely. Bake for 40 minutes, or until a knife inserted in the center comes out clean.

NUTRITION PER SERVING

Calories 140 • Fat 4 g • Fiber 3 g • Protein 3 g • Carbohydrates 25 g

# banana pops

MAKES AS MANY AS YOU HAVE INGREDIENTS FOR

These frozen treats are full of potassium and protein — great nutrients to help your brain to study better! You'll need a double boiler; if you don't have one, you can improvise with a saucepan and a glass bowl that is too big to fit inside the pan, so that it balances on top of the saucepan with its bottom held a few inches above the pan's bottom. You'll also need Popsicle sticks or skewers.

**Bananas**
**Semisweet chocolate chips or bars (peanut butter chocolate chips also work well)**
**Chopped nuts of any kind (peanuts work especially well)**

1. Peel the bananas and cut them in half (widthwise, not lengthwise). Push a Popsicle stick or skewer about 2 inches into the cut end of each banana half. Place the banana pops on a cookie sheet lined with waxed paper and freeze for at least 2 hours.
2. Fill the bottom pan of a double boiler or a saucepan with 2 to 3 inches of water and bring to a boil; then lower the heat so that the water just simmers. If you're using a double boiler, place the upper pan on top of the bottom pan. If you're using a regular saucepan, set in it a glass bowl that rests on the mouth of the pan but doesn't completely fit inside the pan, so that its bottom is suspended just over the simmering water.
3. Place the chocolate in the glass bowl or double boiler and stir just until melted. Watch the chocolate carefully — you don't want it to burn.
4. One by one, dip the frozen bananas into the chocolate mixture, roll them in the chopped nuts, and place them back on the lined baking sheet. Freeze until the chocolate is set. Store in the freezer in ziplock bags.

NUTRITION PER SERVING

Calories 200 • Fat 9 g • Fiber 4 g • Protein 4 g • Carbohydrates 35 g

# coconut rice pudding

MAKES 3 SERVINGS

When you crave dessert, this sweet pudding is easy to whip up.

**½ cup jasmine rice**
**½ cup light coconut milk**
**¼ cup golden raisins**
**4 tablespoons sugar**
**¼ teaspoon cinnamon**
**⅛ teaspoon nutmeg**

1. Cook the rice in a pot on a stovetop according to the package directions, aiming for a slightly firm-textured rice.
2. When the rice has finished cooking, add the coconut milk, raisins, sugar, cinnamon, and nutmeg. Stir over low heat until all of the ingredients are well incorporated and the mixture begins to thicken. Add more coconut milk if necessary to obtain the desired consistency.

NUTRITION PER SERVING
Calories 250 • Fat 10 g • Fiber 2 g • Protein 2 g • Carbohydrates 42 g

# blueberry coffee cake

MAKES 6 SERVINGS

Serve this cake for dessert, then enjoy the leftovers with your morning coffee.

- **Cooking spray**
- **2 tablespoons butter**
- **¾ cup sugar**
- **1 egg**
- **1¼ cups plus 1 tablespoon water**
- **¾ cup all-purpose flour**
- **1 teaspoon baking powder**
- **¼ teaspoon salt**
- **1½ cups blueberries**
- **1 egg yolk**

1. Preheat the oven to 300°F. Lightly grease a pie plate with cooking spray.
2. Cream together the butter and ¼ cup of the sugar in a small bowl.
3. Beat the egg in a large bowl, then add the water. Stir in the flour, baking powder, and salt. Mix in the butter and sugar mixture.
4. Spread the batter in the prepared pie plate. Top with the blueberries.
5. Beat together the egg yolk and the remaining ½ cup of sugar in a small bowl. Sprinkle over the blueberries.
6. Bake for about 35 minutes, until a knife inserted in the center comes out clean.

NUTRITION PER SERVING

Calories 190 • Fat 6 g • Fiber 1 g • Protein 3 g • Carbohydrates 35 g

# gingerbread

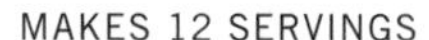
MAKES 12 SERVINGS

A favorite when topped with whipped cream or ice cream.

**Cooking spray**
**1½ cups all-purpose flour**
**2 teaspoons freshly grated ginger**
**2 teaspoons cinnamon**
**1½ teaspoons baking soda**
**1 egg, beaten**
**¼ cup sugar**
**⅓ cup molasses**
**½ cup boiling water**
**¼ cup vegetable oil**
**¼ cup applesauce (see page 235 for our recipe)**

1. Preheat the oven to 350°F. Lightly grease an 8-inch square baking pan with cooking spray.
2. Combine the flour, ginger, cinnamon, and baking soda in a large bowl and mix well. Stir in the egg, sugar, and molasses. Add the water, oil, and applesauce, and mix until the batter is smooth.
3. Pour the batter into the prepared baking pan and bake for about 30 minutes, until a knife inserted in the center comes out clean.

NUTRITION PER SERVING
Calories 150 • Fat 5 g • Fiber 1 g • Protein 2 g • Carbohydrates 24 g

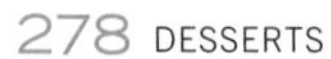

# lemon almond biscotti

MAKES 15 BARS

These cookies keep very well in the freezer.

**Cooking spray**
**1 cup all-purpose flour**
**⅓ cup sugar**
**⅓ cup whole, unblanched almonds**
**1 tablespoon lemon zest**
**½ tablespoon baking powder**
**1 tablespoon vegetable oil**
**1 egg white**
**½ teaspoon vanilla extract**

1. Preheat the oven to 325°F. Lightly spray a baking sheet with cooking spray, then dust with flour.
2. Combine the flour, sugar, almonds, zest, and baking powder in a large bowl. Mix well.
3. Mix together the oil, egg white, and vanilla in a separate bowl. Combine the wet and dry ingredients and stir well. The batter should be sticky.
4. Roll the batter into a log about 1 foot long and place on the prepared baking sheet. Bake for 35 minutes.
5. Remove the log from the oven, and cool for 5 minutes. Leave the oven set at 325°F. Cut the biscotti into ¾-inch slices, and lay the pieces on their sides on the baking sheet. Bake for 10 minutes longer. Cool before serving.

NUTRITION PER SERVING

Calories 60 • Fat 2 g • Fiber 1 g • Protein 2 g • Carbohydrates 10 g

# chocolate soufflé

MAKES 4 SERVINGS

Who would think that we'd include a soufflé in here? The dish is usually thought to be even a professional chef's nightmare. However, we had no trouble with this one. It's made with cocoa mix, which makes things a bit lighter and easier. If you have an electric mixer, you can pull this off easily and people will be impressed. Make sure that you use a large casserole dish with straight sides; the soufflé will rise, so be prepared.

**1 cup skim milk**
**½ cup sugar**
**⅓ cup cocoa mix**
**¼ cup all-purpose flour**
**4 eggs, separated into whites and yolks**
**½ teaspoon cream of tartar**

1. Preheat the oven to 350°F.
2. Combine the milk, ¼ cup of the sugar, the cocoa mix, and the flour in a saucepan, and mix well. Cook over medium heat, stirring constantly, until the mixture has thickened. Set aside.
3. Combine the egg whites and cream of tartar in a large bowl, and beat at high speed until foamy. Continue beating, adding the remaining ¼ cup of sugar bit by bit, until the mixture forms stiff peaks.
4. Stir the egg yolks into the cocoa mixture.
5. Gently fold the chocolate mixture into the egg whites. Pour into an ungreased casserole dish. Bake for 35 to 40 minutes, until the soufflé is puffy and shakes a bit, when the dish is (gently!) moved. Serve immediately.

NUTRITION PER SERVING

Calories 330 • Fat 6 g • Fiber 2 g • Protein 11 g • Carbohydrates 59 g

# peanut butter cookies

MAKES 30 COOKIES

For a little more variety and flavor, try adding some peanut butter chips or chocolate chips to this recipe.

**¾ cup packed brown sugar**
**¾ cup peanut butter**
**4 tablespoons unsalted butter, softened**
**¼ cup applesauce (see page 235 for our recipe)**
**1 teaspoon vanilla extract**
**1 egg, beaten**
**1½ cups all-purpose flour**
**¾ teaspoon baking soda**

1. Preheat the oven to 375°F.
2. Combine the sugar, peanut butter, and butter in a large bowl, and blend well. Stir in the applesauce, vanilla, and egg.
3. Stir together the flour and baking soda in a separate bowl. Gradually add the dry ingredients to the wet ingredients, mixing thoroughly as you proceed.
4. Drop spoonfuls of dough onto an ungreased baking sheet. Gently press each piece of dough with a fork. (Press twice to make a criss-cross pattern.) Bake for about 8 minutes until the cookies are cooked through and beginning to brown on the bottom.

NUTRITION PER COOKIE
Calories 100 • Fat 5 g • Fiber 1 g • Protein 2 g • Carbohydrates 12 g

# oatmeal chocolate chip cookies

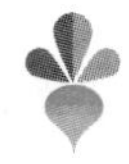

MAKES 24 COOKIES

Two great cookies — oatmeal and chocolate chip — packed into one terrific treat.

- **Cooking spray**
- **½ cup (1 stick) unsalted butter, softened**
- **½ cup packed brown sugar**
- **½ cup granulated sugar**
- **¼ cup applesauce (see page 235 for our recipe)**
- **1 egg, beaten**
- **2 teaspoons vanilla extract**
- **2 cups all-purpose flour**
- **½ teaspoon cinnamon**
- **½ teaspoon salt**
- **½ teaspoon baking soda**
- **1½ cups uncooked quick-cooking oats**
- **1 cup chocolate chips**

1. Preheat the oven to 350°F. Lightly grease a baking sheet with cooking spray.
2. Combine the butter, brown sugar, granulated sugar, applesauce, egg, and vanilla in a large bowl. Mix thoroughly.
3. Combine the flour, cinnamon, salt, and baking soda in a separate bowl. Gradually mix the dry ingredients into the wet ingredients, stirring as you proceed. Stir in the oatmeal and chocolate chips.
4. Drop spoonfuls of dough onto the prepared baking sheet. Bake for 10 to 15 minutes, until the cookies are cooked through and beginning to brown on the bottom. Cool before removing from the cookie sheet.

NUTRITION PER COOKIE

Calories 170 • Fat 7 g • Fiber 0 g • Protein 2 g • Carbohydrates 25 g

# mom's chocolate cake

MAKES 15 SERVINGS

You got us on this one — it's not the least bit healthy. But it does lift the spirits. The secret ingredient is the coffee.

**Cooking spray**
**1¾ cups all-purpose flour**
**2 cups sugar**
**¾ cup cocoa powder**
**2 teaspoons baking soda**
**1 teaspoon baking powder**
**½ teaspoon salt**
**2 eggs, beaten**
**1 cup strong black brewed coffee**
**1 cup skim milk**
**½ cup vegetable oil**
**2 tablespoons lemon juice**
**1 teaspoon vanilla extract**

1. Preheat the oven to 350°F. Lightly grease a 13- by 9-inch cake pan with cooking spray.
2. Combine the flour, sugar, cocoa powder, baking soda, baking powder, and salt in a medium bowl.
3. Combine the eggs, coffee, milk, oil, lemon juice, and vanilla in a separate large bowl. Add the dry ingredients to the wet ingredients and stir. The mixture will look lumpy.
4. Pour the mixture into the prepared cake pan. Bake for about 45 minutes, until a knife inserted in the center comes out clean.

NUTRITION PER SERVING
Calories 250 • Fat 9 g • Fiber 2 g • Protein 4 g • Carbohydrates 41 g

# second edition recipe contributors

**SARAH CAMPBELL**
Terre Haute, Indiana
Indiana State University
*Chicken & Bacon Quesadillas, page 61*
*Slow-Cooked Shredded Italian Beef, page 219*

**CARLA CARDELLO**
North Huntingdon, Pennsylvania
Slippery Rock University
*Peanut Butter Oatmeal, page 26*
*Thai-Inspired Beef and Pasta, page 150*
*Chicken Curry, page 202*

**NANCY DENTLER**
Greensboro, North Carolina
Lamar University alumna
*Crunchy Oatmeal, page 26*
*B.L.T. Tater, page 58*
*Tuna Salad Wrap, page 69*
*Creamy Corn and Potato Chowder, page 86*
*Hoppin' John, page 126*
*Beef 'n' Barley Dinner, page 206*
*Beans 'n' Franks, page 224*

**NANCY ELLIOTT**
Houston, Texas
University of Texas, alumna
*Best Banana-Blueberry Smoothie, page 77*

**TIM EMPRINGHAM**
Burlington, Ontario
Brock University
*Tim's Slow-Cooked Citrus Ribs, page 229*

**SARAH ESKESTRAND**
Denver, Colorado
Truman State University
*Two-Bean Tamale Pie, page 139*

**MARIA FERJANCSIK**
Santa Rosa, California
Sonoma State University
*Lemony Tofu Over Greens, page 129*

**MARY FRENCH**
Cambridge, Massachusetts
Wellesley College
*Lemon-Asparagus Pasta, page 152*
*Roasted Cauliflower, Green Olive, and Almond Pasta, page 156*
*Orecchiette with Broccoli Rabe and Pine Nuts, page 157*
*Spaghetti Squash Marinara, page 237*
*Simple Green Beans, page 239*
*Roasted Beets with Onions, page 243*

**JENNIFER GANDRUD**
Bemidji, Minnesota
Bemidji State University
*Easy Chicken Philly, page 71*

**JES GRAY**
Richmond, Virginia
Virginia Commonwealth University
*Banana Hammer Smoothie, page 77*

**TIMOTHY GUILLOT**
Washington, D.C.
George Washington University
*Bok Choy Salad with Nut-Crusted Chicken, page 107*

**RENEE HAGENS**
Pittsburgh, Pennsylvania
Penn Highlands Community College
*Vegetable and Herb Rice Pilaf, page 248*

**NIKKI HAMBURGER**
Everett, Washington
Art Institute of Seattle
*Slow-Cooker BBQ Ribs, page 228*

**PATRICIA HANCOCK**
Hawthorne, New Jersey
*Toaster-Oven Pita Pizza, page 64*

**DANIEL HARMAN**
Philadelphia, Pennsylvania
Drexel University
*One-Pot Pot Roast, page 222*

**CHRISTOPHER J. HARRIS**
Bloomsburg, Pennsylvania
Pennsylvania College of Technology
*Chicken Caesar Salad with Cranberries, page 101*

**CHARLES HARRIS**
Walla Walla, Washington
Whitman College
*Ginger-Garlic Beef Stir-Fry, page 209*

**JUSTINE HART**
Nashville, Tennessee
University of Iowa
*Slow-Cooked Barbecue Chicken, page 197*

**LOUIS HUFFMIRE**
Anaheim, California
California State University, Fullerton
*Garlicky Olive Chicken, page 199*

**AMANDA KAHN**
San Franciso, California
Suffolk Community College and the Fashion Institute of Technology
*Spinach Pie, page 135*
*Lower-Fat Hummus, page 57*

**PAT KRAIKITTIKUN**
Los Angeles, California
University of California, Irvine
*Spinach Calzone, page 137*

**MARLOWE LEVERETTE**
Columbia, South Carolina
University of South Carolina
*Powered-Up Crispy Treats, page 48*
*Cereal Balls to Go, page 48*
*Fruity-O Smoothie, page 78*
*Green Tea–Melon Smoothie, page 78*

**BRITTANY LUEKEN**
St. Louis, Missouri
Webster University
*Easy Eggplant Pasta, page 153*

**MEGHAN MCKAY**
Poughkeepsie, New York
Marist College
*Meg's Thai Tofu, page 131*

**MARY BETH MCLEES**
Clemson, South Carolina
Clemson University
*Beth's Chicken and Broccoli Bake, page 194*

**PATRICK MCMENAMIN**
Lexington, South Carolina
University of South Carolina
*Slow-Cooker Citrus Salmon, page 175*

**JILL MEHLMAN**
Hamburg, Pennsylvania
Pennsylvania State University
*Slow-Cooker Vegetable Stew, page 120*

**KATHRYN MELLOTT**
Kirksville, Missouri
Truman State University
*Pork Enchiladas, page 226*

**SARA MORRIS**
Dana Point, California
California Polytechnic State University, San Luis Obispo
*Mushroom Pizzas, page 63*

**LAUREN OGLES**
West Monroe, Louisiana
Louisiana Delta Community College
*Chicken Chow Mein Salad, page 106*

**DAWN ONUFFER**
Pittsburg, Pennsylvania
University of Pennsylvania
*Peanut Butter and Banana Smoothie, page 76*

**ROSALIND POPE**
Greensboro, North Carolina
University of South Africa
*Banana–Wheat Germ Smoothie, page 79*

**CAROLE RESNICK**
Iowa State University, alumna
*Chicken Bulgur Salad with Cranberry Vinaigrette, page 114*

**ANNA RICH**
Tuscaloosa, Alabama
University of Alabama
*Spicy Edamame Snacks, page 46*
*Thai Coconut–Red Curry Soup, page 90*
*Salad Caprese, page 103*
*Banana Pops, page 275*

**JEANNETTE RODGERS**
Suwanee, Georgia
Liberty University
*Lemon-Pepper Chicken and Artichokes, page 185*

**EMILY RODRIGUEZ**
Walla Walla, Washington
Whitman College
*Pesto Turkey Sandwich, page 70*
*Green Egg Sandwich, page 75*
*Butternut-Quinoa Soup, page 89*

**ROSIE ROSENBLOOM**
Edison, New Jersey
Queens College
*Asian Chicken Salad Wrap, page 189*

**ANNIE ROSENKRANZ**
Denver, Colorado
Grinnell College
*Quiche-adilla, page 39*
*Mango Salsa, page 253*

**ANINDITA SHABNAM**
Jackson Heights, New York
*Crab-Stuffed Mushrooms, page 49*

**NADA SHAWISH**
Vienna, Virginia
George Washington University
*Italian Chicken Sauté, page 183*

**LISA SKRABAR**
Dunnellon, Florida
Central Florida Community College
*Lime-Basil Mahi Steaks, page 166*

**LEORA STEIN**
Walla Walla, Washington
Whitman College
*African Groundnut Stew, page 122*

**ELANA STONE**
Walla Walla, Washington
Whitman College
*Breakfast Burrito, page 35*

**JONATHAN STRONG**
Las Vegas, Nevada
University of Nevada, Las Vegas
*Mozzarella Grilled Cheese with Tomato and Arugula, page 66*

**ERIC TANNER**
Cincinnati, Ohio
Northern Kentucky University
*Grilled Ham and Roast Beef Sandwich, page 67*

**SARAH TIBBETTS**
Lyman, Maine
University of Maine
*Slow-Cooked Chicken Fiesta, page 191*

**DAWN TODD**
Fayetteville, West Virginia
Kaplan University
*Micki's Roast Turkey, page 223*

**KRISTIN VATTER**
Northfield, Minnesota
St. Olaf College
*Tortellini Soup, page 91*

**JENNY WAGNER**
Madison, Wisconsin
University of Wisconsin, Madison
*Cobb Burger, page 203*
*Sweet Potato Fries, page 246*

**ALLISON WEILER**
Deerfield Beach, Florida
Broward Community College
*Homemade Chinese Takeout, page 188*

**ASHLEY WOLFE**
Williamsport, Pennsylvania
Pennsylvania College of Technology
*Open-Face Quesadillas, page 60*

**HANNAH WOLTERS**
Culleoka, Tennessee
*English Muffin Sundae, page 30*
*Granny's Apple Pie Fruit Salad, page 271*

**KELLIE WUTZKE**
Walla Walla Washington
Whitman College
*Coconut Rice Pudding, page 276*

# index

## c



## d

## n



## o



## p



## q

# other storey books you will enjoy

***The College Cookbook*** **by Geri Harrington**
These two hundred nutritious recipes will save the busy — and often broke — college student.
160 pages. Paper. ISBN 978-0-88266-497-2.

***Dorm Room Feng Shui*** **by Katherine Olaksen**
This introduction to feng shui for the college student has
practical tips for clearing the chi in every dorm room.
144 pages. Paper. ISBN 978-1-58017-592-0.

***Raw Energy in a Glass*** **by Stephanie Tourles**
Best-selling author Stephanie Tourles offers more than 120 super-nutritious, super-delicious recipes for smoothies, shakes, green drinks, power shots, mocktails, and fermented beverages, all designed to boost your health and energy. All of the recipes can be made in a standard blender.
288 pages. Paper. 978-1-61212-248-9.

***Soup Night*** **by Maggie Stuckey**
Bring the neighborhood together with your own soup night and 90 crowd-pleasing recipes for hearty chowders, chili, and vegetable soups for every time of year. Additional recipes for salads, breads, and dessert round out the soup night experience.
304 pages. Paper. 978-1-61212-099-7.

**Storey BASICS® Series: Cooking**
The essential information you need to get things done. With titles such as *How to Make Ice Cream*, *Knife Skills*, and *Making Vegan Frozen Treats*, Storey Basics are the ideal resource for any beginner or seasoned cook looking to expand their skills. These portable, highly accessible guides, written by experts, provide the perfect amount of information to ensure success right from the start.
Paper. Learn more about each title by visiting *www.storey.com.*

***Ultimate Dining Hall Hacks*** **by Priya Krishna**
Make the most of your college meal plan with this inventive cookbook. Using 100 basic foods available in any college dining hall, put together 75 delicious main courses and snacks, including Chicken and Cheese Quesadillas, Greek Pizza, Peach Cobbler, and plenty more.
128 pages. Paper. ISBN 978-1-61212-450-6.